POWER
SOUPING

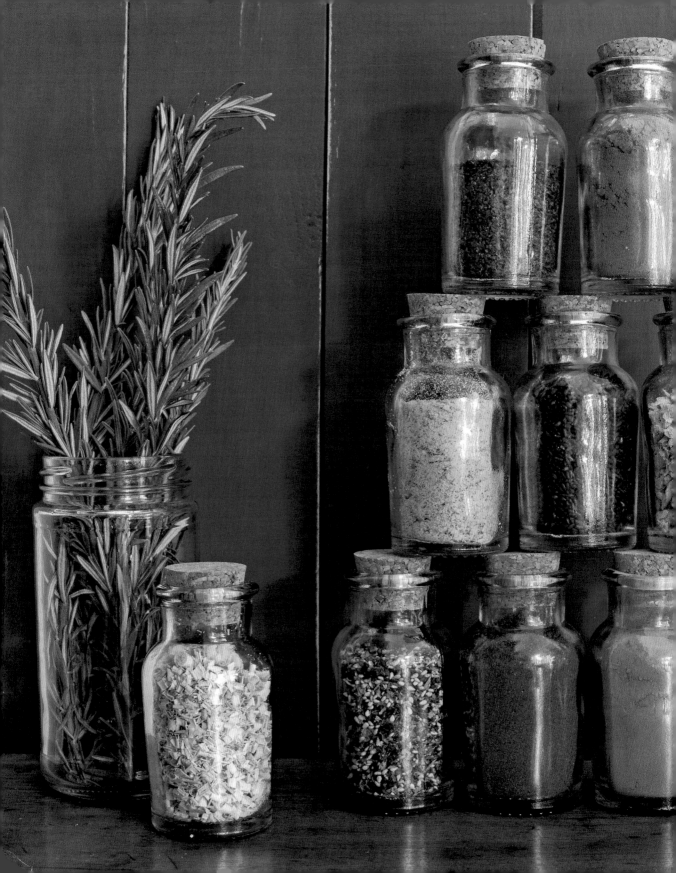

POWER SOUPING

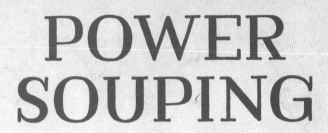

3-DAY DETOX, 3-WEEK WEIGHT-LOSS PLAN

Rachel Beller, MS, RDN

WILLIAM MORROW

AN IMPRINT OF HARPERCOLLINS*PUBLISHERS*

ALSO BY RACHEL BELLER

EAT TO LOSE, EAT TO WIN

The health advice presented in this book is intended only as an informative resource guide to help you make informed decisions; it is not meant to replace the advice of a physician or to serve as a guide to self-treatment. Always seek competent medical help for any health condition or if there is any question about the appropriateness of a procedure or health recommendation.

HarperCollins books may be purchased for educational, business, or sales promotional use. For information please e-mail the Special Markets Department at SPsales@harpercollins.com.

FIRST EDITION

Design by Kris Tobiassen / Matchbook Digital

Linen background photograph by ©iStock.com Andrea Astes

All other photographs by Teri Lyn Fisher except for photographs on pages ii–iii, vi, viii, 4, 15, 18, 74–75, 98, 104, 138, 141, 146, 156, 167, 192, 198–199, 208–209, 211, 213, 218, 236, 242, and 244–245 by Nicole LaMotte

Library of Congress Cataloging-in-Publication Data has been applied for.

ISBN 978-0-06-242492-1

16 17 18 19 20   ID/QG 10 9 8 7 6 5 4 3 2 1

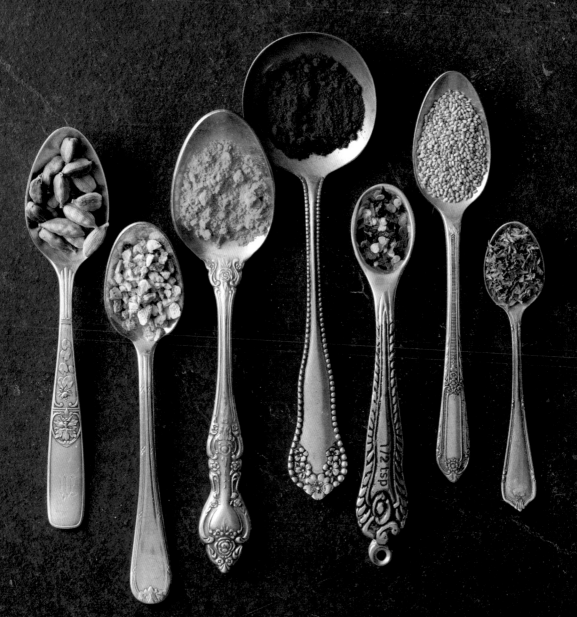

To my parents, my four kids, and my husband,

THE LOVING FORCES OF MY LIFE; FOR PUTTING A SMILE ON MY FACE EACH AND EVERY DAY; WHO IS MY BEST FRIEND

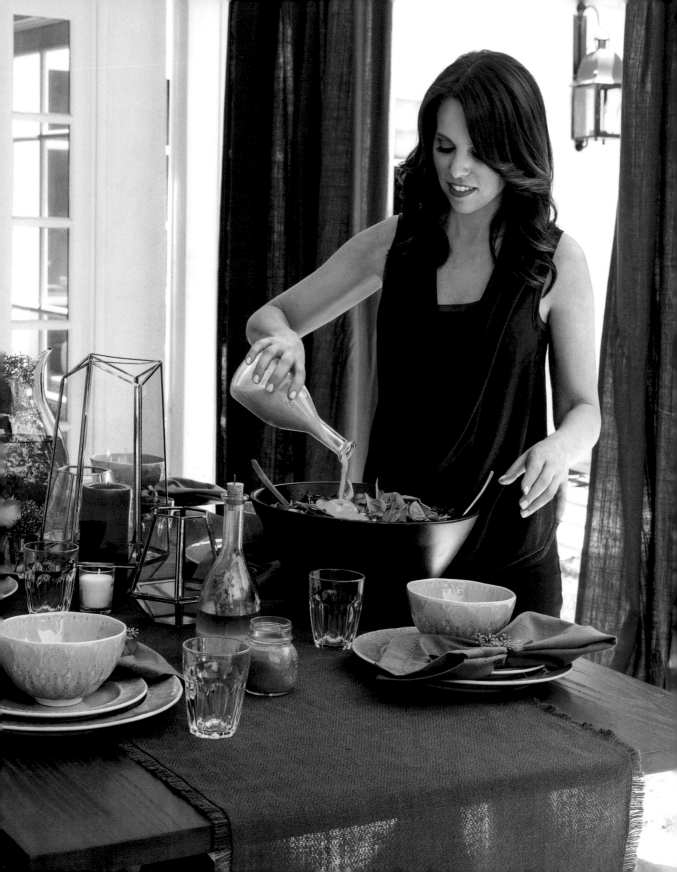

CONTENTS

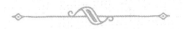

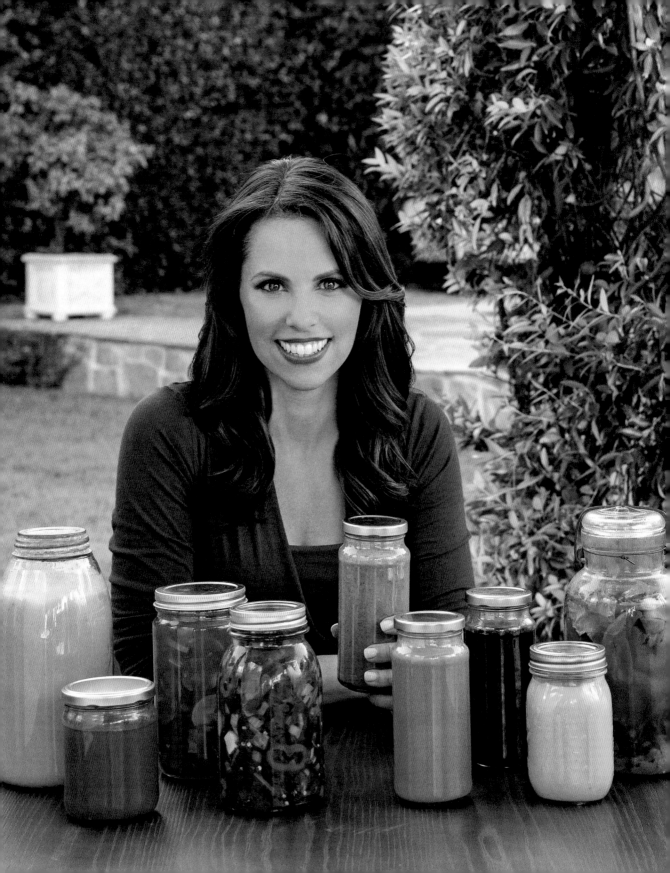

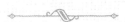

THE SOUPING LIFESTYLE

Souping has never been hotter.

I don't mean temperature or spice (though the more spices the better)! I'm talking about how anyone looking to lose weight and detox these days—from working moms to movie stars to CEOs—is getting their soup on. In fact, souping is the new juicing—only *better*! And I'll tell you why.

My office is in Beverly Hills—which is ground zero for juicing. Every other person on the street is clutching a bottle of some apple–kale–lawn clipping concoction. And I totally see the appeal of this type of diet. People want something quick and easy and with strict parameters. They like being boxed into drinking what's in that bottle—and that's it. No room for error.

But I can't tell you how many of those people wind up in my office because they're miserable, starving, have no energy and Just. Need. Something. Else. *Please!*

That's because while juice diets are billed as "cleanses" or "detoxes," the one ingredient with the most detoxing power—fiber—is trashed after the juice is squeezed out, often leaving you with sugar water. Sounds crazy, but it's absolutely true. Plus, most of them don't have nearly enough protein to keep you satiated.

Take a look.

Detox Juicing

The Marketing Department Needs to Clean Up Its Act

For those of you who aren't familiar with my Food Autopsies, they're a deep dive inside foods that appear healthful but actually aren't—like this popular "cleansing" juice. Hollywood types are willing to fork over ten dollars for a small bottle of this stuff!

But what they don't know is that they're guilty of a DUI—**d**rinking **u**nder the **i**llusion that anything green in a fancy bottle is good for you.

Here's the crime: The front of the bottle lists amazing ingredients, such as kale, spinach, romaine, parsley, cucumber, celery, apple, and lemon, along with the words "100% Juice" in big letters. It makes you think you're getting an entire salad through a straw.

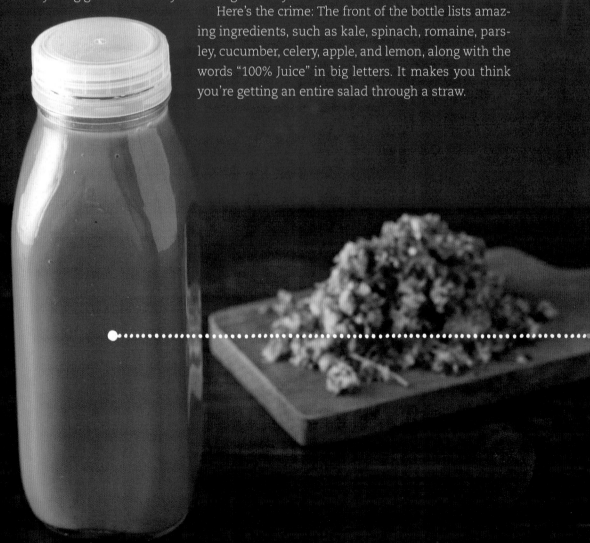

Now spin that bottle around and take a closer look at the label, because the first ingredients you see listed make up the bulk of the juice. This is what you're *really* getting: apple juice (first and foremost), then small amounts of juices from cucumber, celery, romaine lettuce, lemon, spinach, kale, and parsley leaf. Notice that the most nutrition-rich juices are at the very end—and their intensely green flavor has been strategically masked in sugary apple juice. I call this "green-tinted liquid candy."

In fact, this one bottle of "detox" contains 28 grams of sugar, but *none* of the full, natural fibers the produce originally came with. That's one bad combo! With no fiber to blunt the natural sugars in the juice, what you're really paying for is a ticket on a blood-sugar roller-coaster ride that will have you feeling hungry again in no time. That's not a real cleanse—it's your wallet getting cleaned out. Can we talk felony here?

If you truly wanted a cleanse, you'd ask for all the stuff they tossed after the "juicing": the pulp, peels, and leaves. That's where you'll get the most of the valuable fiber and nutrients. It's like throwing away nutritional gold!

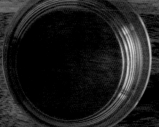

**SHOT OF
VEG JUICE**

**GLASS OF
APPLE JUICE**

As a nutrition expert who has helped people lose countless pounds, I know that fad diets don't work—and not just because they're unsatisfying or nutritionally weak. The biggest reason they fail is that once the diet's over, there's no plan about what to do next. Without maintenance guidelines, people fall back into old eating habits and regain the weight. This plan has you 100 percent covered here with a realistic maintenance strategy.

Souping: A Lifestyle, Not a Trend

Here's what makes this plan *soup-erior* to juice diets and other cleanses and detox plans. Souping is:

1. **Cleansing.** Souping is *real* detox, containing all the nutrients you need in one bowl. I'm talking health-boosting antioxidants, fiber, protein, and good-for-you omega-3 fats to naturally cleanse your insides and keep you satisfied.

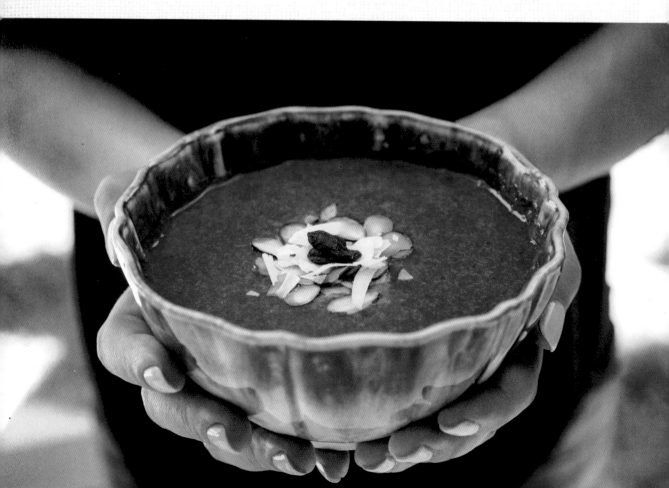

2. Controllable. The thing people love about juicing is the calorically set meals—one bottle and done. No extras. And that's one thing souping shares with this type of plan. You have a single bowl—one that actually contains real, filling, yet still low-cal food—and you're set. That's why so many studies have linked soup with weight loss and maintenance. (You can read more about that on page 238.)

3. Comforting. Soups taste and feel like real meals, because they are. They've got everything you need—vegetables, protein, healthful fats, and wholesome carbohydrates—and you can't think soup without also thinking comfort. And that makes souping sustainable, because it doesn't feel like a capital-D diet chore.

4. Convenient. Making a big pot of soup and taking single servings with you to work—or having leftovers as a ready-to-go dinner—is easy and economical. No more scrambling to fetch the right fast bite or overpaying for a tiny bottle of juice that's going to leave you hungry in 20 minutes.

Commit to 3 days of straight souping, and you'll reboot your body and lose around 3 pounds. (I'll show you how in Chapter 2.) And that's just to get you started! After the 3 days, you'll embark on a 24-Day Transformation plan that combines soups and plated meals. (I lay all that out in Chapter 3.) Once you've lost the weight and are feeling recharged, it's time for Maintenance mode (Chapter 4). I'd never hold your hand and then let go at the end! So I'll show you simple strategies that will help you keep the weight off for good. Finally, in Chapter 5, I'll answer all of your questions, let you in on the science behind souping—yes, there's a ton of research showing it works—and give you the scoop on some of my nutrition recommendations.

Soup's on! But before you dig in, I'd like to show you why I want you to stick *only* to the soups in this book (at least for now) and not stray into the wild world of prepared options. Because not any old bowl will do.

Food Autopsies: Meet—but Don't Eat—the Wrong Soups

Turn the page and let me dissect four *souper* common misconceptions for you.

The "Healthful" Smoothie Bowl

Big Toppings Make for Big Bottoms
(and Not in a Sexy, Kim Kardashian Way)

Let's begin by taking a look at the hottest thing in morning meals on Instagram right now: decked-out smoothie and acai bowls, a.k.a. "breakfast soups."

Most smoothie bowls start off right with a balanced base of fruit and other clean foods (250 to 300 calories, on average). That is not the problem—it all goes south when we get to the toppings.

My CSI (**c**aloric **s**candal **i**nvestigation) reveals that these beautiful smoothie bowls are topped off with some mega unintentional calories. A major offender: granola (code for belly-expanding cookie crumbs) is usually chock-full of added sugar and can end up tipping the scale in the wrong direction.

So, while I love smoothie and acai bowls, I'm calling *time-out* on the topping overload.

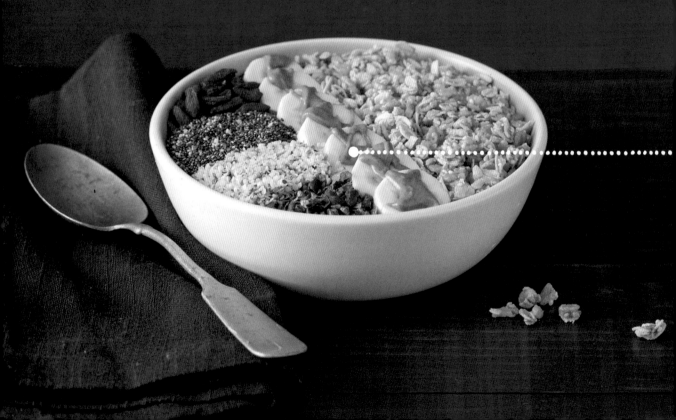

HERE'S A LOOK INSIDE A TYPICAL INSTAGRAM SMOOTHIE BOWL POST:

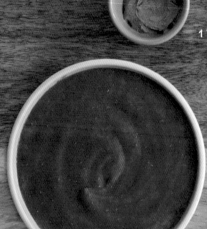
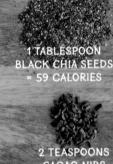

1 TABLESPOON
ALMOND BUTTER
= 96 CALORIES

1 TABLESPOON HEMP SEEDS
= 53 CALORIES

⅓ CUP GRANOLA
= 173 CALORIES

1 TABLESPOON
BLACK CHIA SEEDS
= 59 CALORIES

1 TABLESPOON
GOJI BERRIES
= 33 CALORIES

2 TEASPOONS
CACAO NIBS
= 28 CALORIES

1 LARGE BANANA
= 120 CALORIES

TOPPING TOTAL = 562 CALORIES!
+ 300 CALORIES FROM THE SMOOTHIE BOWL BASE

862 CALORIES TOTAL!

The smoothie bowl plus the topping insanity means *you are starting your day with a whopping 800 to 850 calories.* Yes, they are calories from clean foods—but as real as they may be, they're capable of packing on real pounds.

Don't worry! I designed all my smoothie bowls to allow for these tasty toppings, but I've kept the calories in line so that you'll size down, not up!

FOOD AUTOPSY:
"Convenient" Canned Soup

Veggie-Less Salt Water

Now let's examine a popular brand of canned soup. After all, it's a convenient and popular all-American staple that's marketed as a cheap, easy, and healthful way to get dinner on the table.

The downsides? An almost complete lack of vegetables—I'm not convinced those tiny orange cubes even count as carrots. And the insanely refined noodles are equivalent to nearly 2 slices of fiberless white bread! Another problem? Salt, salt, and more salt!

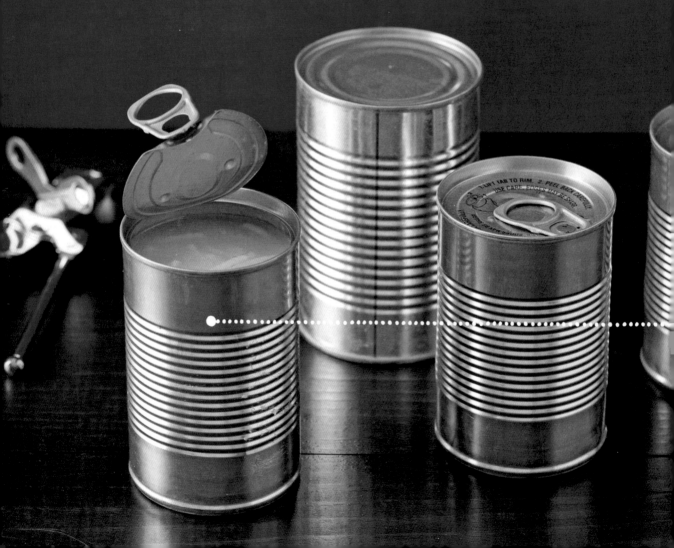

An average can of a popular condensed chicken noodle soup has 2,350 milligrams of sodium—more than most adults should consume in an entire day. Too much sodium in your diet can lead to belly bloat and, more important, a laundry list of other health problems.

So what, exactly, are you eating? It's almost as if you're slurping salt water with chunks of soggy bread and über-processed bits of chicken. As if all of that weren't bad enough, your classic chicken noodle soup contains MSG, chicken fat, and Frankenfood soy isolates.

The takeaway here is this: No matter how cheap and easy store-bought soup may seem, if you're getting nothing out of it, it's still a rip-off!

A better option? One of my No-Brainer Soups on pages 118–120. They take minutes to make, are wallet friendly—and contain, yes, *actual nutrition*.

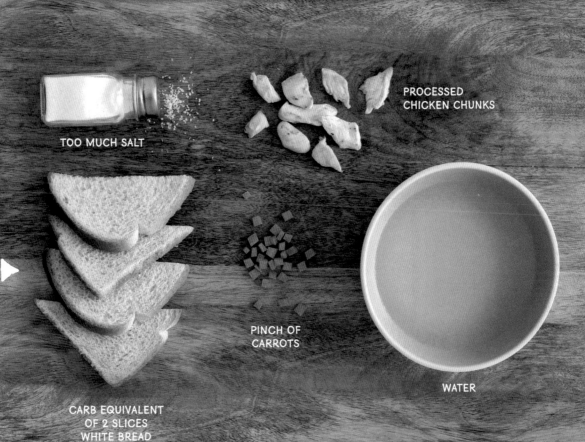

TOO MUCH SALT

PROCESSED
CHICKEN CHUNKS

PINCH OF
CARROTS

WATER

CARB EQUIVALENT
OF 2 SLICES
WHITE BREAD

FOOD AUTOPSY:
Packaged Ramen Noodles

They Shouldn't Even Be Called "Food"

Everyone knows the contents of those packets and foam cups are far from nutritional wonders. But if you read the label, you'll be horrified. It's worse than you thought. Let's take a quick look.

Noodle Ingredients

Enriched wheat flour: Don't be fooled by the word "enriched"—it's code for processed white flour.

TBHQ: (a.k.a. tert-butylhydro-quinone) Dare you to say that three times fast! This is a preservative that has been linked to nausea, tinnitus, vomiting, and tumor incidence. *Mmmm.*

Soup Base Ingredients

Monosodium glutamate, or MSG: This notorious flavor enhancer has been known to cause headaches, sweating, nausea, and chest pain in some people. No thanks!

Maltodextrin: A texturizer made from heavily processed corn, potato, rice, or wheat starch—ingredients that used to be real foods but are now more chemical than anything else.

Hydrolyzed corn, wheat, and soy protein: Chemically broken-down (think dropped in a vat of sulfuric acid, boiled, then neutralized with lye), low-quality proteins.

Disodium inosinate: A chemical added to *enhance* the potency of MSG—as if it weren't potent enough already!

Natural flavors: Exactly what are these, anyway? Maybe long ago they hailed from natural sources, but after intense processing in a lab, they're definitely not natural anymore.

There are even more impossible-to-pronounce ingredients, but if I were to explain them all, this would become a chemistry textbook. There's no real food to be found anywhere. How we survived on ramen in college is a mystery!

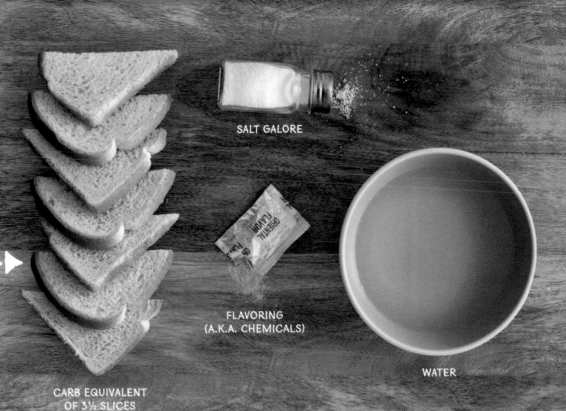

SALT GALORE

FLAVORING
(A.K.A. CHEMICALS)

WATER

CARB EQUIVALENT
OF 3½ SLICES
WHITE BREAD

FOOD AUTOPSY:
Restaurant Noodle Bowls

Hide Your Eyes!

It may seem safer to order noodle soup from one of those gourmet ramen joints—but it isn't much better. The ingredients may be fresher, but don't let them deceive you. Here's my perception-beats-deception trick: Take your twelve-dollar ramen home and let it cool in the fridge. When you take it out, you'll see this congealed beige lump emerging from the bowl. What you're looking at: a fat bomb.

And it gets worse. I went ahead and dove into that mess—from one of the most popular ramen joints in L.A.—and here's what I found.

First, you'll overdose on processed carbs—the noodle carbs equal 5 slices of white bread per bowl! And what exactly is the "soup" that those empty carbs are drowning in? Try melted lard. I counted 6 *tablespoons* of solid fat in my sample. As for veg, there's a single depressing tablespoon of chives—that's it. Now let's do another CSI:

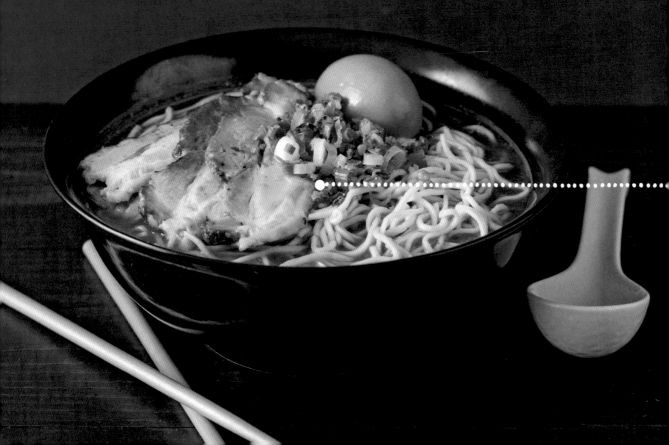

2½ cups of noodles = 400 calories
This is what most dieters should have per meal alone.

6 heaping tablespoons of pork fat = 600 calories
You heard me—pork fat! You're getting 600 calories just from lard!

Chashu pork slices = 200 calories
¼ pound of thick slices of salty bacon braised in soy sauce, sugar, and sake.

Soft-boiled egg = 70 calories
I like eggs, but I don't like them soaked in salt-loaded soy sauce.

Total calories = 1,270

So you're essentially eating 2½ orange-tinted lard sandwiches that contain no fiber or vegetables—and consuming nearly 1,300 calories along the way.

Here's a better idea: If noodle bowls are your thing, check out my veggie-and-protein-packed pho on page 227. You'll get all of the satisfying slurp you need.

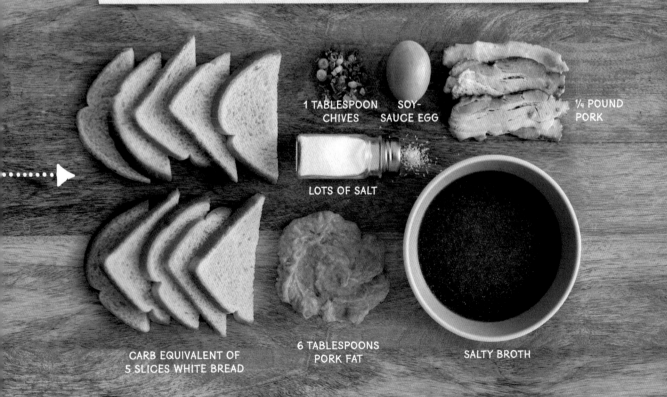

1 TABLESPOON CHIVES

SOY-SAUCE EGG

¼ POUND PORK

LOTS OF SALT

CARB EQUIVALENT OF 5 SLICES WHITE BREAD

6 TABLESPOONS PORK FAT

SALTY BROTH

The *Right* Soups

The soups in this book don't leave out essentials like whole, fiber-rich vegetables, which fill you up and take your antioxidant intake from minimal to supercharged! In my fifteen years of conducting research and working with clients, I've found that plant-based meals are the way to go for both weight loss and health. All of the recipes in this book include a base that's rich in essential nutrients straight from Mother Nature. Plus, my signature Power Up toppers (herbs, spices, powerfoods) can further boost your immunity and overall health while making your meal extra flavorful. My souping plan is designed around the same foundational principles that I use in all of my fast-track weight-loss methods—whether they involve a spoon or a fork.

Souping checks off all of the nutritional boxes I value most:

☑ Fiber? Check!

☑ Antioxidants? Check!

☑ Protein? Check!

☑ Essential fats? Check!

☑ Easy? Check!

☑ Tasty? Check!

☑ Affordable? Check!

☑ Satisfying? Check!

☑ Cleansing? Check!

☑ Effective? Check!

In fact, I'm so convinced that souping works, I don't just recommend it to my clients—I'm a power souper myself.

So grab a spoon and get ready to soup!

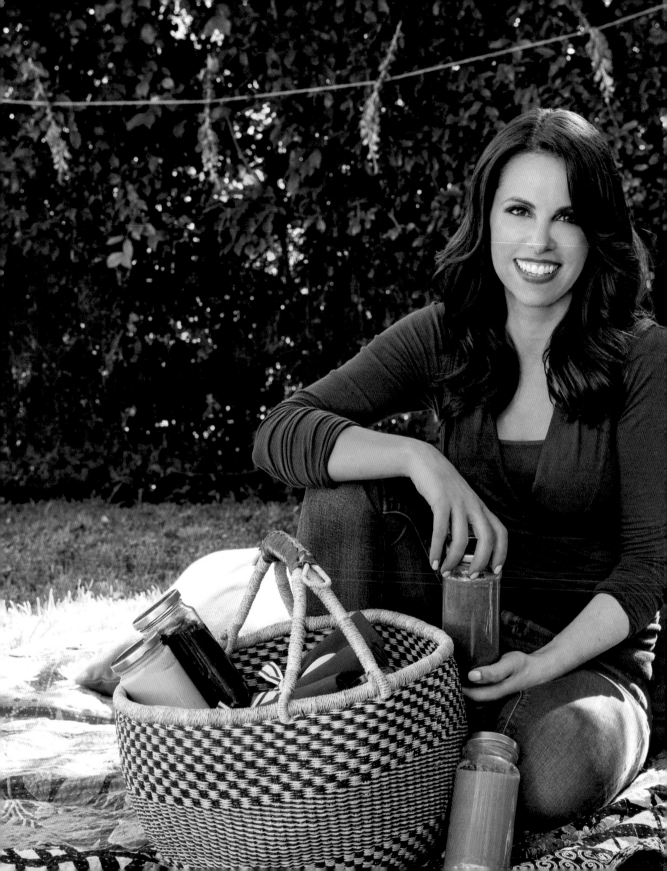

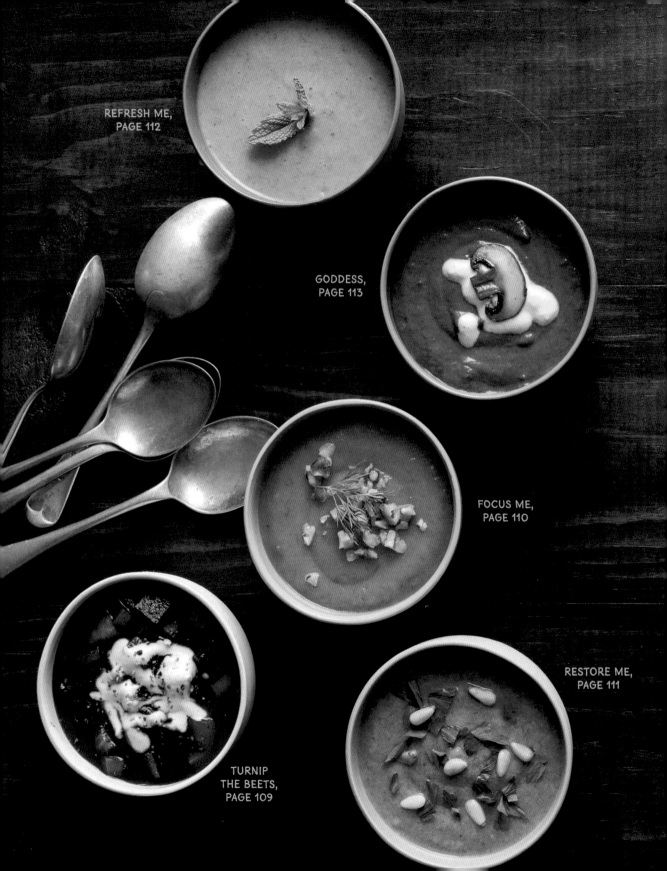

REFRESH ME,
PAGE 112

GODDESS,
PAGE 113

FOCUS ME,
PAGE 110

RESTORE ME,
PAGE 111

TURNIP
THE BEETS,
PAGE 109

1.
Nourish Me

❦

ALL THE RECIPES YOU NEED
FOR WEIGHT-LOSS SUCCESS
AND SOUP-ERIOR HEALTH

From breakfast smoothie bowls to savory dinner soups, this chapter is loaded with all of the easy-to-make recipes you'll need for the 3-Day Restart as well as the 24-Day Transformation. You'll even find Freebie Soups (clean, detox-y, and super low-cal) that you can enjoy anytime, especially when you need a little extra. The majority of the soups are vegan and gluten-free and use a wide variety of wholesome, real ingredients. You'll also find my favorite Power Up powerfood toppers.

Enjoy!

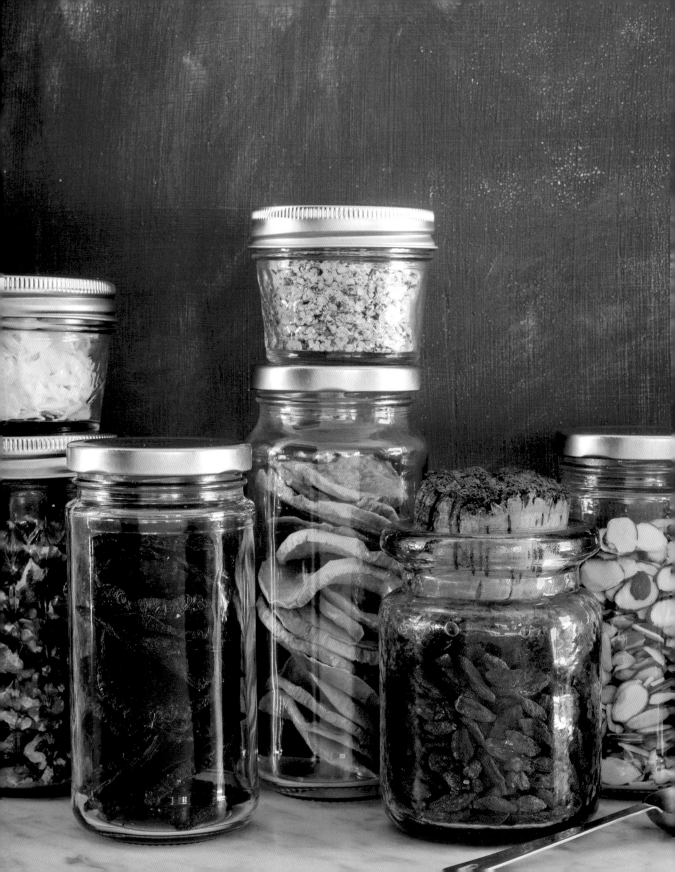

Fridge and Pantry Basics

You don't need any fancy or expensive equipment to soup. But there are a few fridge and pantry staples that are good to have on hand because you'll be using them again and again during all parts of my plan. Read on and stock up!

Beans: Pick up a variety of them, like chickpeas, cannellini, and black beans. Soaking and cooking dried beans is the best way to prepare them—check out my how-to on pages 140–141. But the realist in me knows that's not always doable in our busy lives. The next best option is to buy them in Tetra Paks (see Chapter 5 for more information). I like the Whole Foods 365 Everyday Value brand and Target Simply Balanced.

Broth (low sodium): Making broth from scratch—either bone broth or veggie—is ideal from a flavor and freshness standpoint. However, I totally get the need for convenience! There are tons of premade choices out there, but a couple of brands I prefer are Pacific Foods and Imagine Foods. When picking a broth, look for varieties with less than 140 milligrams of sodium per serving, that are organic, have no MSG, and come in a BPA-free container such as a Tetra Pak.

Ceylon cinnamon: Not all cinnamon is the same! About 90 percent of the cinnamon sold in the United States is cassia cinnamon, a type with higher levels of coumarin—a chemical that may cause liver toxicity if ingested in excess. Ceylon cinnamon is *true* cinnamon. It's a healthier alternative that may also offer antioxidant and blood-sugar-control benefits. It also has a lighter, sweeter flavor compared to cassia cinnamon.

Chia seeds: These fiberlicious seeds are widely available in supermarkets and health stores alike. They come in black and white varieties—but it's not the color that lends to their nutritional value. Instead, look for seeds that are similar in size and shape. This uniformity is a good indication that the seeds are grown in one region and yield a consistent nutritional value.

Dates: They're among the sweetest fruits around—so just one date goes a long way to delivering lots of flavor along with nutrients and fiber.

Frozen bananas: Save yourself the stress of trying to eat them before they go brown! Instead, peel and freeze them just before they ripen (more resistant starch, less sugar) and you'll have a constant supply. It's an easy way to thicken, sweeten, and cool down your breakfast soups.

Ghee: This type of clarified butter delivers an intensely rich and buttery taste, so just a small amount goes a long way. Ghee has a high smoke point, making it ideal for high-heat cooking. Additionally, the way that ghee is produced makes it a great alternative if you have any kind of dairy intolerance.

High-quality oils: My go-to for almost everything is extra-virgin olive oil. Whichever oil you choose, be sure to buy it in a dark glass bottle and store it in a cool, dark place to prevent spoilage. Different oils have varying smoke points, so it's important to use the right oil for the job! Here's a quick rundown:

Unrefined, cold-pressed extra-virgin olive oil: It has a strong flavor, greenish color (from chlorophyll pigments), and a low smoke point, so it's best for salads, dressings, and cold dishes.

Refined extra-virgin olive oil: With a relatively high smoke point, this oil is best for medium- to high-heat cooking, such as baking, braising, or a gentle sauté.

Extra-light olive oil: This light-colored olive oil has a high smoke point, so it's good for high-heat cooking like broiling, grilling, stir-frying, and roasting. And it has a neutral taste that won't affect the flavor of your dish.

Avocado oil: It adds a slight buttery avocado flavor to foods and has a very high smoke point that makes it suitable for high-heat cooking and searing. Bonus: It's also rich in heart-healthful monounsaturated fats!

Walnut oil: With a rich, nutty taste, it's high in omega-3 fatty acids. While you can use it for medium-heat cooking, walnut oil's flavor is best showcased in cold dishes and salads.

Coconut oil: Coconut oil is a rich source of medium-chain triglycerides. These kinds of fats are rapidly metabolized for immediate energy. Go for the virgin variety, which is less refined and has more antioxidants than other types. Use coconut oil for medium-heat cooking.

Kefir: Found in the dairy section next to the yogurts, this drinkable probiotic superstar has tons of nutritional benefits. Both cow and goat kefir are available, but I prefer goat. Be sure to select the plain, unsweetened, organic types to avoid added sugars, and choose 2% (reduced fat) instead of full fat or nonfat. If you can't find 2%, 1% is okay (see Chapter 5 for more information).

Legumes: Hailing from pod-producing plants, legumes are packed with resistant starch and protein. Good sources that do not require soaking before cooking include lentils (red, brown, and green) and split peas (green and yellow). Sprouted is preferred for maximum nutrient value and absorption.

Maple syrup: Grade A Dark Color is my favorite because it packs a big flavor punch—so you can use less and still get the sweetness you crave in a totally all-natural form. It's still sugar but has a leg up from refined sugar, because it's relatively unprocessed and contains some naturally occurring minerals.

Matcha: These green tea leaves come in a fine powder. Be sure to buy the ceremonial grade—which should have a vibrant green hue, smooth texture, and mild sweet flavor—not the cooking grade, which has a coarser consistency and bitter taste. You can find it at health food stores and online.

Mung beans: A tasty comfort food that can be found in grocery and health food stores dried in bags, these beans don't require any soaking before you cook them. If available, buy the sprouted kind for easier digestibility and superior nutrition.

Nuts: I'm talking about the raw, unsalted kind. They don't need to be doused in salt to be delicious!

Nut butters: Choose natural, organic nut butters that require refrigeration after you open them. The conventional kinds contain unnecessary extras like added sugars, hydrogenated oils, and preservatives for longer shelf life. Make sure the only ingredients are nuts and maybe a little salt. You'll need to stir in the oil layer on top—but that separation is natural and a sign that your nut butter is the real deal.

Nutritional yeast: This is a favorite among vegans because it's chock-full of essential B vitamins and adds a nutty, cheesy flavor. You'll find it online or at any health food store. Nutritional yeast comes in powdered and flaked forms—both of which yield the same result.

Organic miso: Miso is a thick, savory paste made from fermented soybeans that imparts a rich, salty flavor to many types of dishes (especially soups!). You can find miso in health food stores and some supermarkets in the refrigerated section.

Plant-based milks (unsweetened): These are vegan, mild, and waistline-friendly—and will serve as the base for many of your breakfast soups, so stock up! While homemade milks are best (see my recipe on page 139), the realist in me gets that making them yourself is not always an option. So just make sure to buy the plain, unsweetened varieties that don't have any added sugars, thickeners, or preservatives. Some of my favorites are almond, cashew, coconut, and hemp milks.

Plant-based protein powder: My favorites are vegan and organic because they're usually cleaner in terms of ingredient sourcing. What makes a "clean" protein powder? Look for products that don't contain chemicals, sugars (of any kind), artificial flavors, super-processed soy or whey isolates, or hydrogenated anything. My go-to brands include Vega One, Sunwarrior, and Garden of Life.

Precut frozen fruits and vegetables: These are major time savers for your breakfast smoothies and soups! And frozen fruits and veggies can be more nutritious than fresh—they're picked at their peak ripeness and immediately frozen, locking in nutrients that are sometimes lost during transit of fresh produce. Bonus: Financially, frozen produce is a great deal, even if you go organic!

Psyllium husk: Loaded with soluble fiber, this powder may lower cholesterol levels, ease digestion, and control your appetite, research has shown. It supplies a thick, viscous texture to your smoothie bowls. Find psyllium husk in any supermarket or health food store.

Raw honey: Studies suggest that this filtered, unpasteurized honey may have antibacterial, anti-inflammatory, immune-boosting, and antioxidant properties. Despite all of its health benefits, it's still a sweetener and should be used sparingly.

Salt: I prefer to season with sea salt or pink Himalayan salt because they're obtained naturally from the sea and undergo minimal processing. They still possess all their healthful essential minerals and may contain a smaller amount of additives than your typical table salt.

Sprouted, organic tofu: You can find this plant-based protein in pretty much any grocery store these days, but be sure to always go for the organic option. When possible, buy sprouted because it has a higher nutrient profile and is easier to digest.

Tamari (reduced sodium): This is a gluten-free version of soy sauce that has a darker color and more complex, smooth flavor than traditional soy sauce. Always try to find a lower-sodium version!

Tomato paste: Buy this souping essential in a jar to avoid BPA.

Vegan yogurt: Even though it is made from plant-based milks, it still contains health-promoting probiotics like traditional yogurt. I like the unsweetened cultured coconut milk yogurt from So Delicious, but there are other types available. Just make sure to buy the plain, unsweetened kind. Of course, you can also make my Vegan Yogurt (page 135) substitution at home.

Wakame: Edible, nutritious seaweed comes in many forms and this variation has a slightly salty taste. Just a small bit adds a ton of flavor. Find this sea vegetable dried in a health food store.

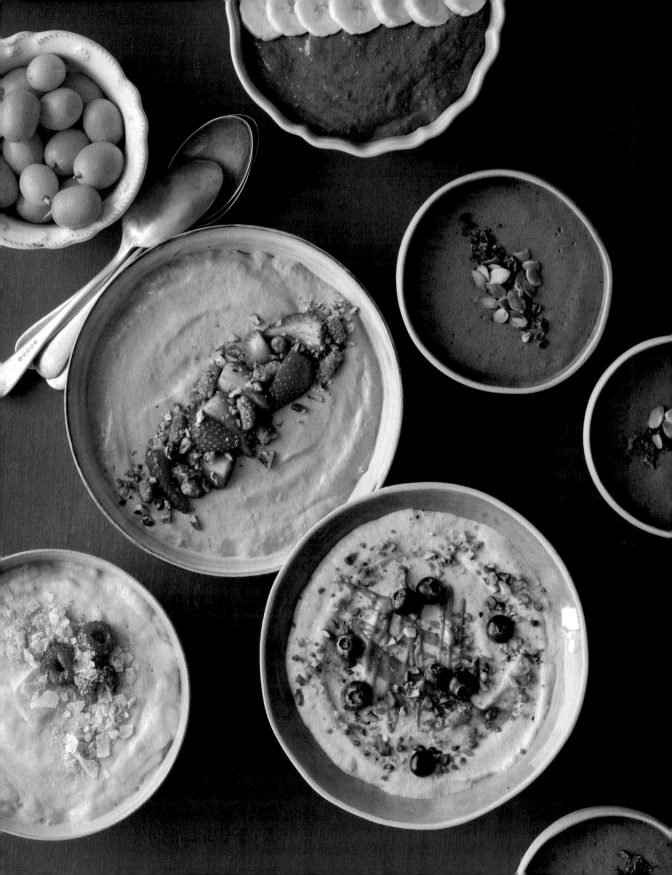

Breakfast

※

I get it, A.M.s can be absolute madness, so I've made these nutrition-loaded recipes super easy to follow. Each of these breakfast soups is full of detoxing fiber and antioxidants, takes just minutes to make, and is totally portable. You can customize them to your tastes by dressing up the naked base with power-packed toppings that amp up the flavor and nutrition of your morning meal (see page 56 for my Power Up toppers). Turn the page for my carefully constructed breakfast soups and learn how to DIY the right way on page 54.

RACHEL'S MORNING RUSH TIPS:

- Preload your blender cup the night before with all ingredients except the liquid. In the morning, simply pour in your liquid, blend, add toppings, and go.

- Keep a lineup of your favorite dry toppings in jars with a measuring spoon so you can easily toss them on.

- If bananas aren't your jam, substitute frozen avocado slices, frozen mango chunks, or plant-based-milk ice cubes.

Shine: MANGO BERRY

MAKES 1 SERVING

VO *Vegan option*   **GF** *Gluten-free*

½ cup unsweetened plant-based milk (see page 139)

¼ cup organic plain 2% Greek yogurt, Vegan Yogurt (page 135), or ¼ avocado

1 cup frozen mango chunks

½ cup frozen strawberries

½ cup frozen raspberries

1 teaspoon chia seeds

OPTIONAL TOPPINGS

2 teaspoons ground flaxseed

2 tablespoons diced mango

Imagine breakfast in a tropical paradise, and this dish comes pretty close! (Beach sold separately.) With its bright boost of vitamin C, it's actually as sweet for your body as it is for your taste buds.

So when those summer mornings hit—or when you want to make a winter morning as bright as possible—greet the day with a bowl of sunshine.

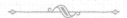

Place the milk, yogurt, mango, strawberries, raspberries, and chia seeds in a high-powered blender and puree until smooth. Dress with toppings, if desired.

MEAL MATH per serving			*Toppings add* 32 calories; 2g fiber			
calories	*fat*	*sodium*	*carbs*	*fiber*	*sugar*	*protein*
240	5g	130mg	42g	11g	31g	10g

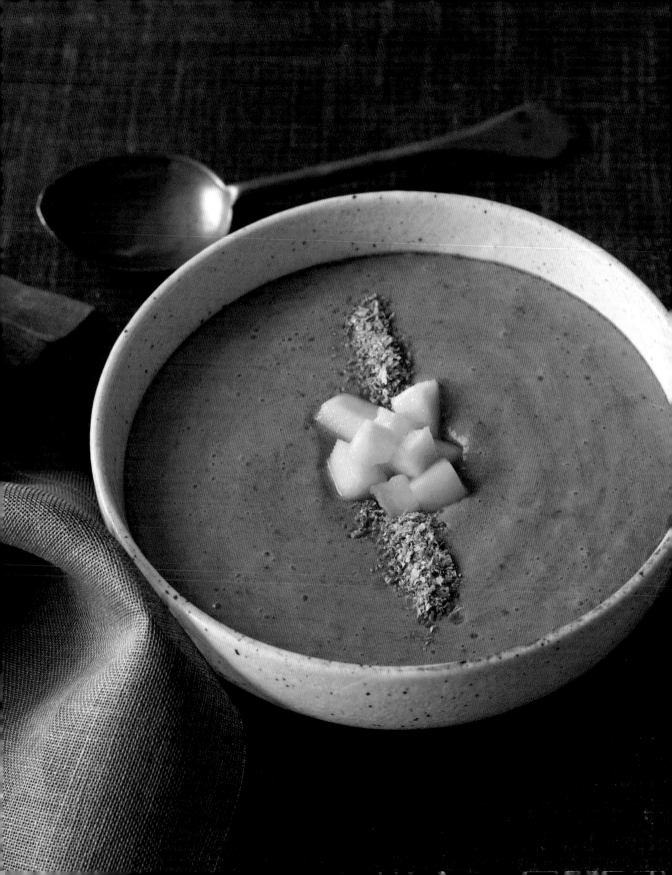

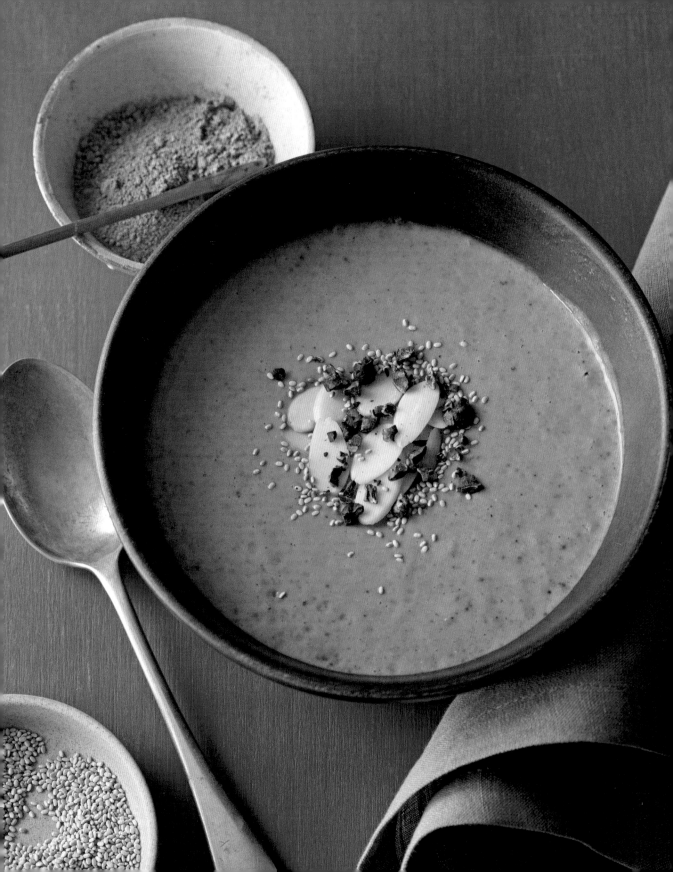

Bliss Me:
MATCHA GREEN TEA

MAKES 1 SERVING

V Vegan   GF Gluten-free

Matcha rules in my book. Made of green tea leaves, matcha not only is a potential weight-loss warrior but it also contains up to 137 times more EGCG (epigallocatechin gallate) antioxidants than normal green tea, which may help you battle harmful free radicals. And since you're also starting your day with the matcha-based A.M. riser, this smoothie bowl guarantees you get a double dose of it.

1 cup unsweetened plant-based milk (see page 139)

1 small frozen banana

1 teaspoon matcha powder

1 tablespoon chia seeds

¼ teaspoon Ceylon cinnamon

½ teaspoon granulated orange peel (optional)

OPTIONAL TOPPINGS

1½ tablespoons sliced almonds

1 teaspoon chia seeds

1 teaspoon raw cacao nibs

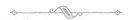

Place the milk, banana, matcha powder, and chia seeds in a high-powered blender and puree until smooth. Sprinkle with cinnamon to taste and the orange peel, if using. Dress with toppings, if desired.

MEAL MATH per serving			Toppings add 84 calories; 4g fiber			
calories	fat	sodium	carbs	fiber	sugar	protein
190	8g	230mg	26g	11g	12g	6g

Radiance: CARROT CAKE

MAKES 1 SERVING

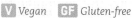 Vegan **GF** *Gluten-free*

¾ cup unsweetened plant-based milk (see page 139)

1 small frozen banana

1 tablespoon plant-based protein powder

1 cup chopped carrots

½ teaspoon Ceylon cinnamon

1 tablespoon chia seeds

2 ice cubes

1 date, pitted (optional)

OPTIONAL TOPPINGS

2 teaspoons chopped walnuts

1 teaspoon raisins

1 teaspoon shredded carrot

Sprinkle of Ceylon cinnamon

You wouldn't dare eat cake for breakfast, right? (Though many people do—they just call it "bran muffins.") On the flip side, you probably wouldn't crave a cup of chopped carrots in the morning. But with this immunity-boosting breakfast soup, you can have your cake—and eat it, too!

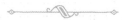

Place the milk, banana, protein powder, carrots, cinnamon, chia seeds, ice cubes, and, if using, the date in a high-powered blender and puree until smooth. Dress with toppings, if desired.

MEAL MATH per serving			*Toppings add* 41 calories; 0g fiber			
calories	*fat*	*sodium*	*carbs*	*fiber*	*sugar*	*protein*
310	11g	310mg	47g	15g	24g	18g

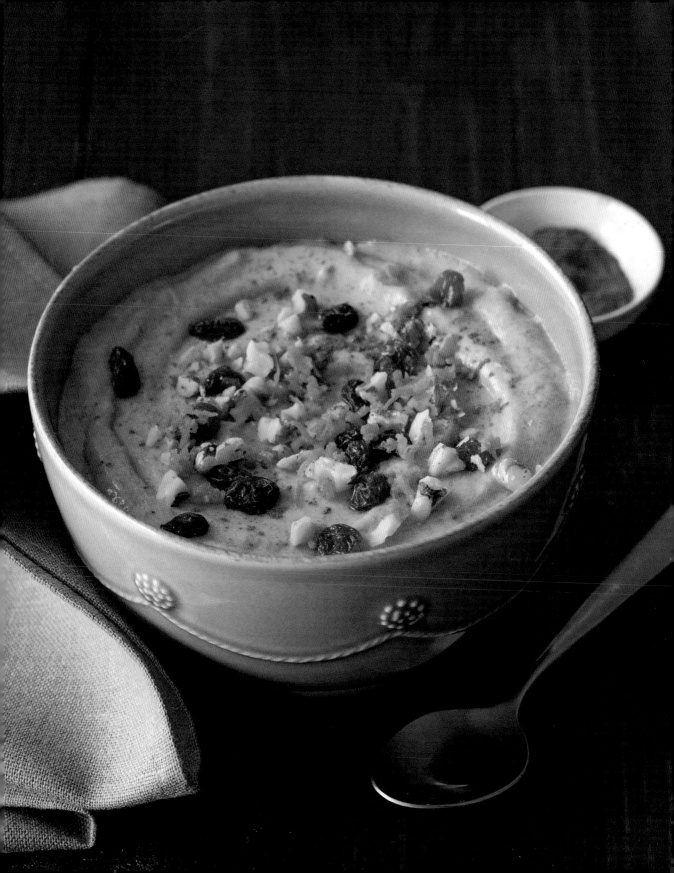

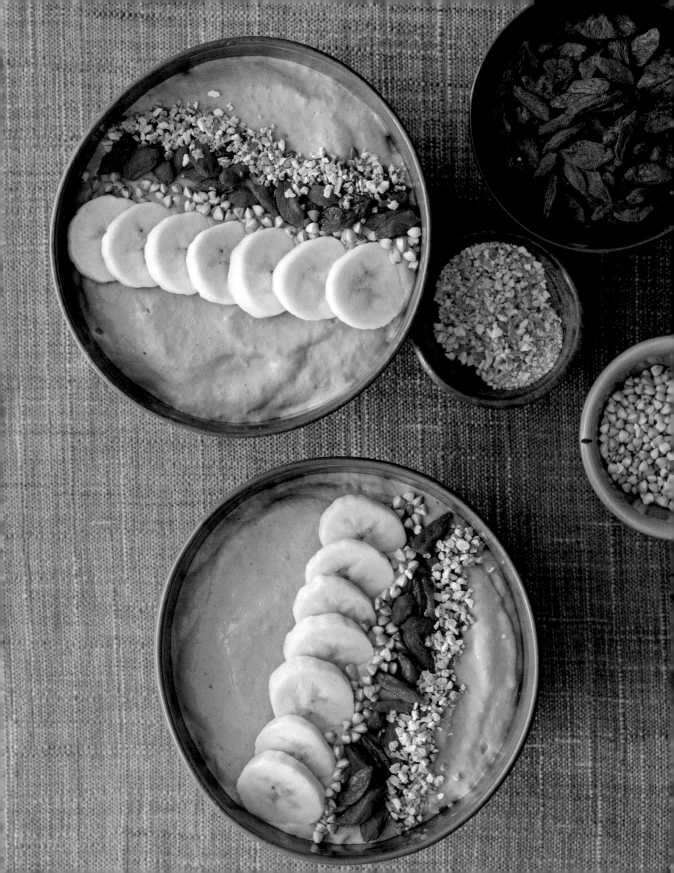

The Beller Basic:
SIMPLE GREENS

MAKES 1 SERVING

VO *Vegan option* **GF** *Gluten-free*

I usually assign this soup to nutrition newbies since they're not used to gazing at a bowl of green first thing in the morning. It's simple, fast, and easy—but it's no nutritional lightweight!

It's boosted with kefir, so treat yourself to a taste sensation that's creamy, tart, and has three times more probiotics than yogurt.

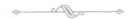

Place the banana, kefir, spinach, cinnamon, and chia seeds in a high-powered blender and puree until smooth. Dress with toppings, if desired.

½ small banana, sliced

½ cup organic plain 2% kefir, unsweetened plant-based milk (see page 139) or Vegan Yogurt (page 135)

1 cup baby spinach

¼ teaspoon Ceylon cinnamon

1 tablespoon chia seeds

OPTIONAL TOPPINGS

2 teaspoons chopped pecans

1 teaspoon buckwheat groats

1 tablespoon goji berries

MEAL MATH per serving			*Toppings add* 122 calories; 2g fiber			
calories	fat	sodium	carbs	fiber	sugar	protein
220	6g	130mg	31g	10g	18g	11g

Indulge Me:
RASPBERRY RED VELVET

MAKES 2 SERVINGS (SERVING SIZE: 1 CUP)

V Vegan **GF** *Gluten-free*

½ cup unsweetened plant-based milk (see page 139)

½ small frozen banana, or ⅓ avocado

1 tablespoon plant-based protein powder

2 small red beets, peeled, raw or steamed

1 cup frozen raspberries

3 tablespoons raw cacao nibs

1 tablespoon peanut butter or other nut butter

2 dates, pitted (optional)

OPTIONAL TOPPINGS

1½ teaspoons raw cacao nibs

2 tablespoons unsweetened coconut flakes

3 raspberries

Here's everyone's favorite sweet-tooth satisfier: beets! (Not what you were expecting, right?) Beets might be the last ingredient you'd expect in a "red velvet cake," but in this recipe, you'll love them. Both beets and raspberries have loads of phytochemicals that help neutralize toxins in your body. Along with ingredients like creamy peanut butter, dates, plant-based protein powder, and crunchy raw cacao nibs, this is one healthful breakfast that you'll actually crave.

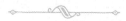

Place the milk, banana, protein powder, beets, raspberries, cacao nibs, peanut butter, and dates in a high-powered blender and puree until smooth. Dress with toppings, if desired.

MEAL MATH per serving				Toppings add 73 calories; 2g fiber		
calories	fat	sodium	carbs	fiber	sugar	protein
240	13g	130mg	29g	13g	12g	12g

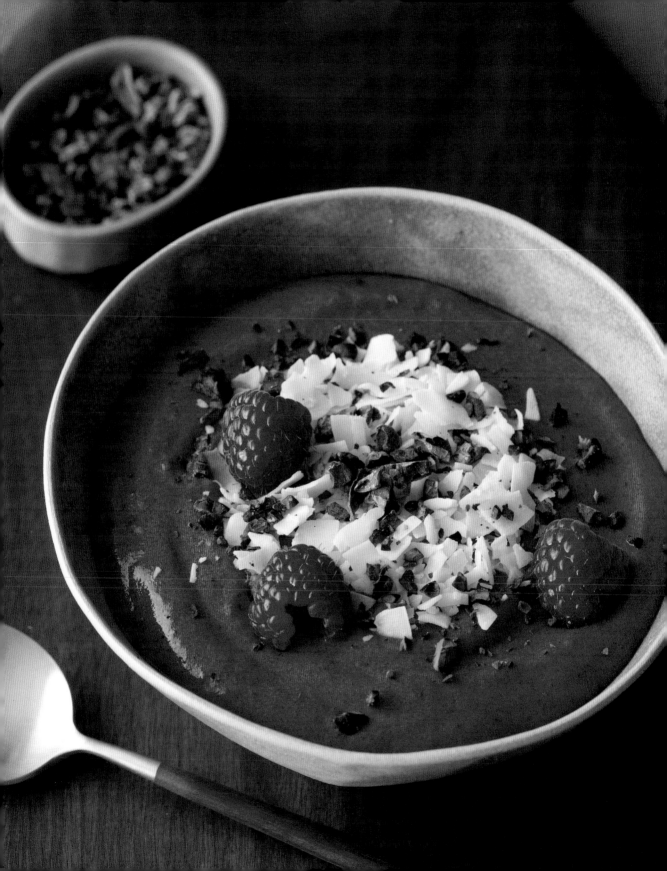

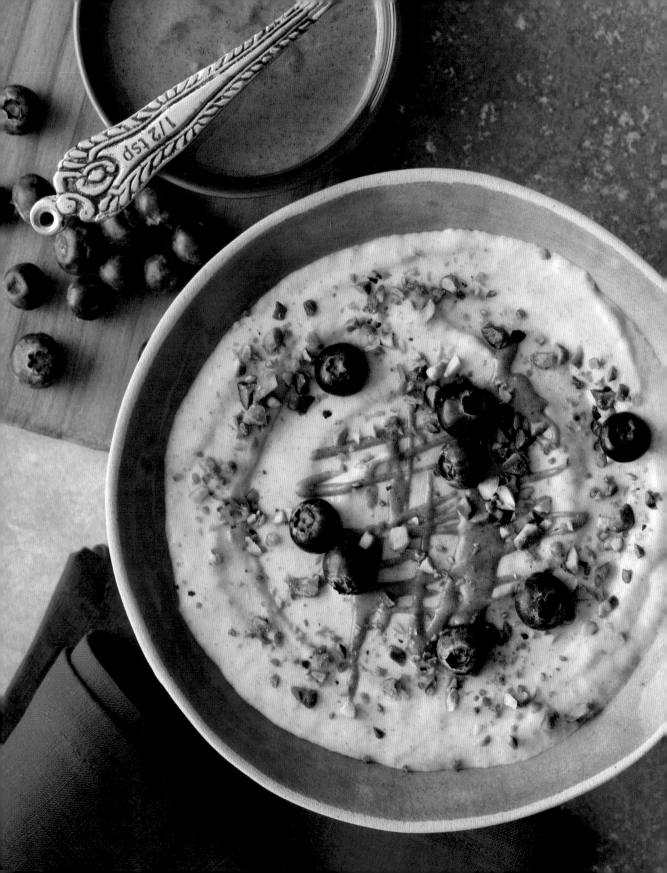

Detoxi-Pie Me:
CREAMY ALMOND PEACH PIE

MAKES 1 SERVING

V Vegan **GF** Gluten-free

This delicious smoothie bowl reminds me of that oh-so-comforting pie usually on the table around the holidays—but with a nutritious edge. Creamy almond butter, spices, and peaches come together for a surprisingly rich breakfast soup that's sweet as pie—without all the added sugar that comes with it.

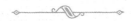

Place the milk, almond butter, peaches, cinnamon, chia seeds, ice cubes, and, if using, the pumpkin pie spice and maple syrup in a high-powered blender and puree until smooth. Dress with toppings, if desired.

1 cup unsweetened plant-based milk (see page 139)

2 teaspoons almond butter

1 cup frozen peaches

¾ teaspoon Ceylon cinnamon

1 tablespoon chia seeds

2 ice cubes

¼ teaspoon pumpkin pie spice (optional)

1 teaspoon pure maple syrup (optional)

OPTIONAL TOPPINGS

1 teaspoon almond butter

2 teaspoons chopped pistachios

8 blueberries

MEAL MATH per serving			Toppings add 66 calories; 1g fiber			
calories	fat	sodium	carbs	fiber	sugar	protein
260	16g	200mg	20g	10g	13g	7g

Treat Me:
CHOCOLATE BANANA

MAKES 1 SERVING

V Vegan   **GF** Gluten-free

½ cup unsweetened plant-based milk (see page 139)

1 tablespoon plant-based protein powder

½ medium banana or ½ avocado

14 whole raw almonds or 1 tablespoon almond butter

2 tablespoons raw cacao powder

4 ice cubes

1 date, pitted (optional)

OPTIONAL TOPPINGS

1 teaspoon rolled oats

1 teaspoon pepitas

½ medium banana, sliced

I don't know what it is about chocolate and banana, but together, they're magic. And this smoothie bowl is no exception. With 2 whole tablespoons of pure raw cacao, you're giving your body a powerful anti-inflammatory boost while getting your chocolate fix, too. If you're craving a creamy bowl of ice cream with toppings, then start your blender!

Place the milk, protein powder, banana, almonds, cacao powder, ice cubes, and, if using, the date in a high-powered blender and puree until smooth. Dress with toppings, if desired.

MEAL MATH per serving			*Toppings add* 72 calories; 2g fiber			
calories	fat	sodium	carbs	fiber	sugar	protein
280	16g	110mg	28g	10g	8g	20g

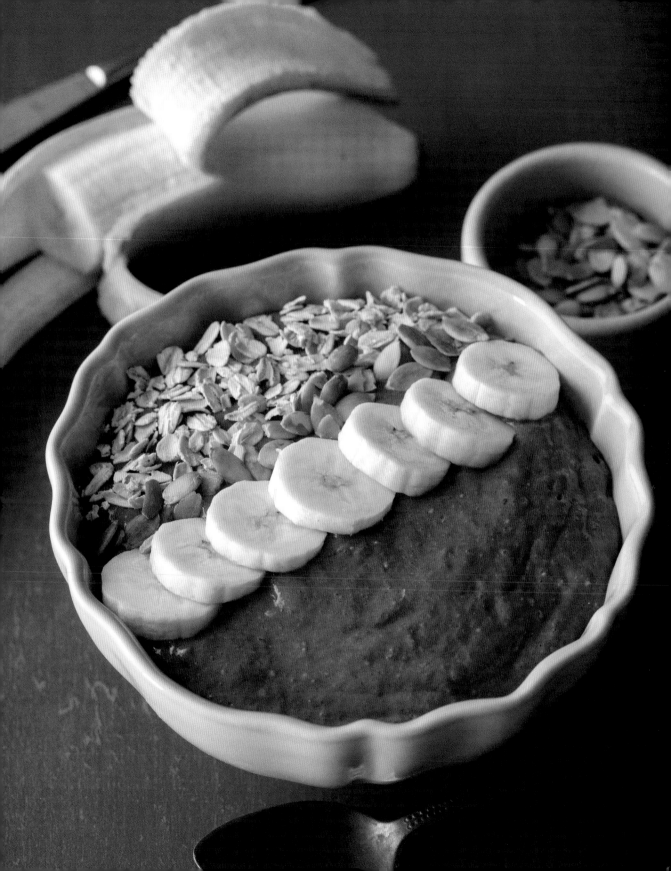

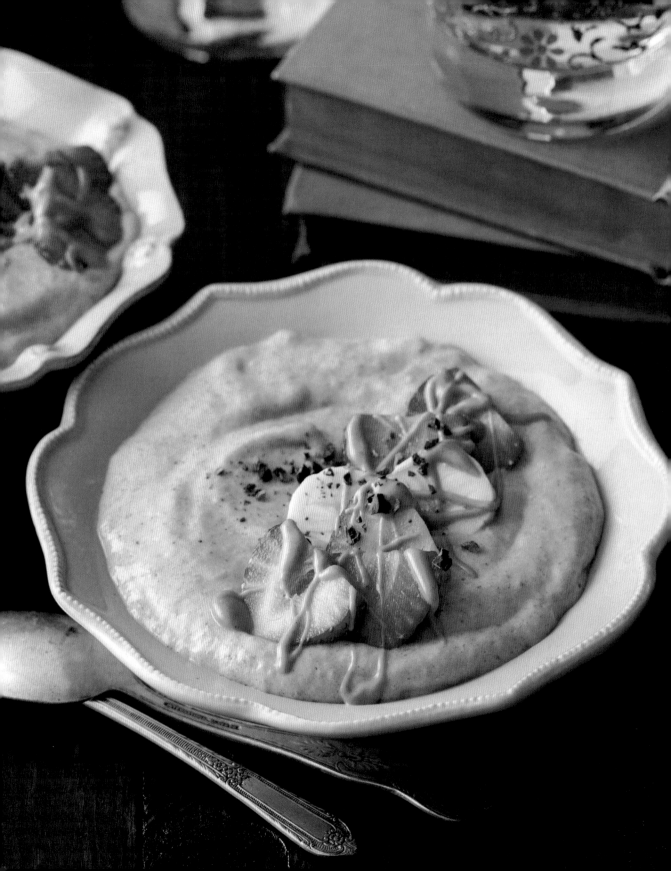

Inner Child:
PEANUT BUTTER AND JELLY

MAKES 1 SERVING

VO *Vegan option* **GF** *Gluten-free*

Bring out your inner child with this revamped peanut butter and jelly bowl. This isn't your old-fashioned crustless sandwich—this smoothie gets you a third of the way to your daily fiber goal and replaces that sugary jam with fresh fruit.

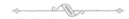

Place the milk, yogurt, banana, strawberries, peanut butter, chia seeds, and ice cubes in a high-powered blender and puree until smooth. Dress with toppings, if desired.

¼ cup unsweetened plant-based milk (see page 139)

¼ cup organic plain 2% Greek yogurt or Vegan Yogurt (page 135)

1 small frozen banana

¾ cup fresh sliced strawberries

2 teaspoons peanut butter

2 teaspoons chia seeds

3 to 4 ice cubes

OPTIONAL TOPPINGS

1 strawberry, sliced

2 slices banana

1 teaspoon peanut butter

½ teaspoon raw cacao nibs

MEAL MATH per serving				Toppings add 55 calories; 3g fiber			
calories	fat	sodium	carbs	fiber	sugar	protein
290	11g	100mg	38g	10g	22g	12g

Balance Me:
BERRIES AND GREENS

MAKES 1 SERVING

 Vegan GF Gluten-free

1 cup filtered water

1 small frozen banana

3 frozen strawberries

½ cup frozen blueberries

2 cups baby spinach

2 teaspoons almond butter

2 teaspoons chia seeds

OPTIONAL TOPPINGS

1½ tablespoons R. B.–approved Spiced Buckwheat Granola (page 137)

1 strawberry, sliced

This nourishing breakfast soup has strawberries, blueberries, banana . . . and spinach. Yes, spinach—and a heavy dose of it, too! With the addition of almond butter and chia, you're getting your protein, antioxidants, and a whoppin' 12 grams of fiber before you even head out the door.

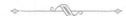

Place the filtered water, banana, strawberries, blueberries, spinach, almond butter, and chia seeds in a high-powered blender and puree until smooth. Dress with toppings, if desired.

MEAL MATH per serving			Toppings add 74 calories; 1g fiber			
calories	fat	sodium	carbs	fiber	sugar	protein
270	10g	90mg	42g	11g	23g	8g

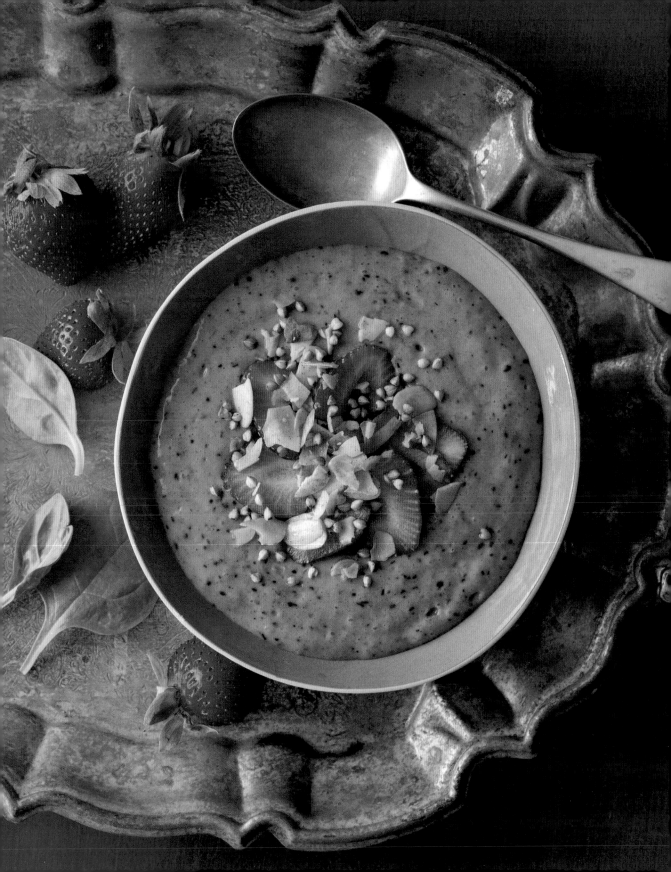

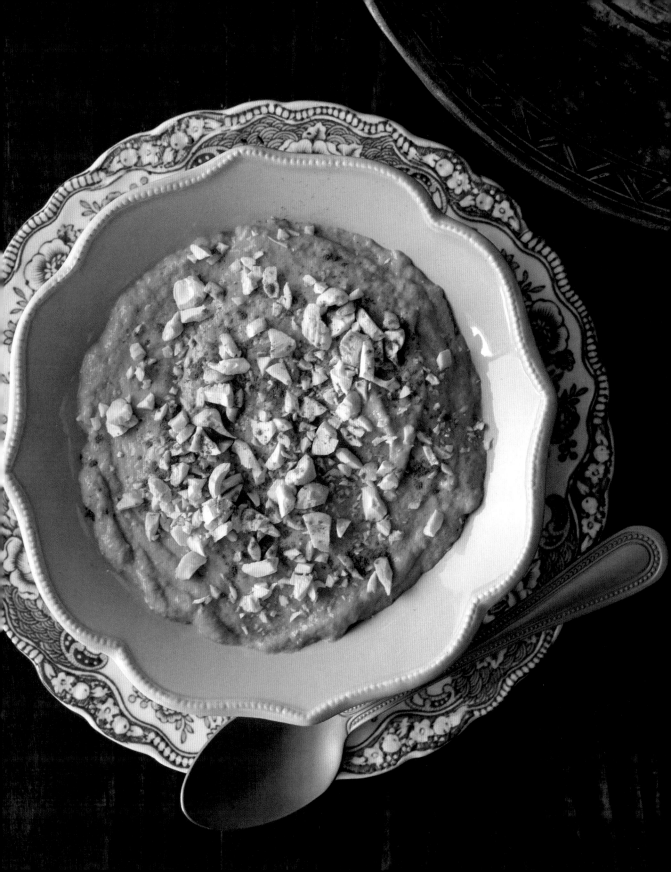

Glowing Green:
SWEET GINGER KALE

MAKES 1 SERVING

VO *Vegan option* **GF** *Gluten-free*

What you feed your body at the beginning of your day should be energizing and fresh. Supercharge your morning routine with ginger—one of the most potent anti-inflammatories around! And don't let the bright green color throw you off—all the fiber in kale will scrub your insides squeaky clean so you glow from the inside out.

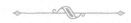

Place the milk, yogurt, banana, kale, ginger, chia seeds, cinnamon, turmeric, and, if using, the honey in a high-powered blender and puree until smooth. Dress with toppings, if desired.

⅓ cup unsweetened plant-based milk (see page 139)

¼ cup organic plain 2% Greek yogurt or Vegan Yogurt (page 137)

1 small frozen banana

½ cup chopped fresh or frozen kale

½-inch piece fresh ginger, peeled and minced

1 tablespoon chia seeds

¼ teaspoon Ceylon cinnamon

¼ teaspoon peeled and minced fresh turmeric or ⅛ teaspoon ground (optional)

1 teaspoon raw honey (optional)

OPTIONAL TOPPINGS

1 tablespoon chopped raw cashews

Sprinkle of Ceylon cinnamon

MEAL MATH per serving			*Toppings add* 49 calories; 0g fiber			
calories	fat	sodium	carbs	fiber	sugar	protein
230	7g	140mg	30g	10g	15g	12g

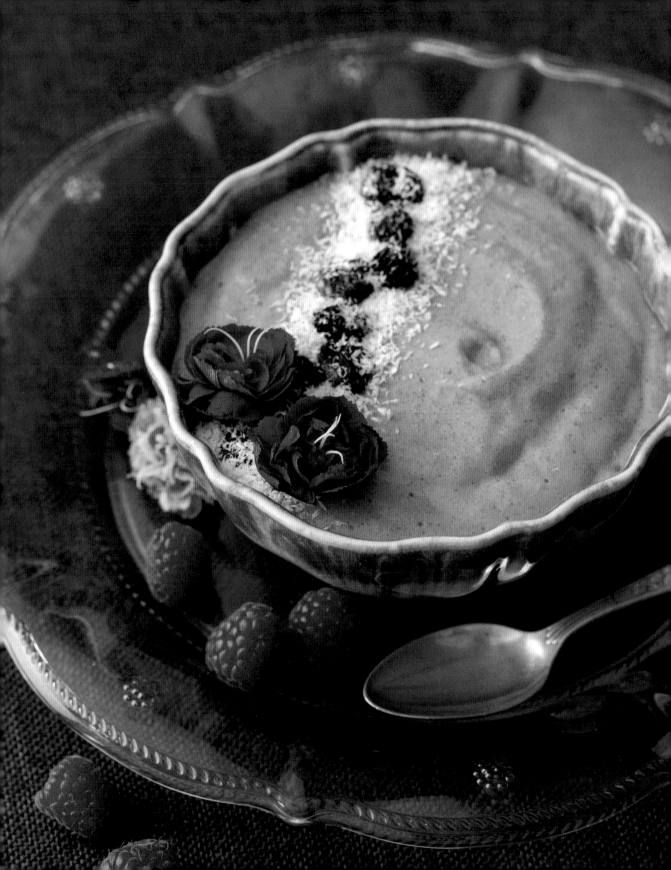

Flawless:
RASPBERRY PEACH

MAKES 1 SERVING

V *Vegan* **GF** *Gluten-free*

Wake up and feel flawless with this fruity breakfast soup. Raspberries are packed with skin-brightening vitamin C and gut-scrubbing fiber that will make you feel radiant and cleansed. Plus, studies suggest that these berries, with their healthful dose of ellagic acid, may fight skin, lung, and breast cancers.

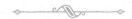

Place the coconut water, raspberries, chia seeds, peaches, protein powder, ice cubes, and, if using, the maple syrup in a high-powered blender and puree until smooth. Dress with toppings, if desired.

1 cup unsweetened coconut water

1 cup frozen raspberries

1 tablespoon chia seeds

½ cup sliced frozen peaches

1 tablespoon plant-based protein powder

4 ice cubes

1 teaspoon pure maple syrup (optional)

OPTIONAL TOPPINGS

2 teaspoons dried golden berries

2 teaspoons unsweetened coconut flakes

MEAL MATH per serving			*Toppings add* 34 calories; 1g fiber			
calories	*fat*	*sodium*	*carbs*	*fiber*	*sugar*	*protein*
260	10g	340mg	34g	19g	18g	19g

Deflame Me:
GINGER, COCONUT, AND TURMERIC

MAKES 1 SERVING

V Vegan   GF Gluten-free

½ cup unsweetened
coconut milk

1 small frozen banana

1 tablespoon plant-based
protein powder

2 teaspoons almond butter

½-inch piece fresh turmeric,
peeled and minced, or
½ teaspoon ground

½-inch piece fresh ginger,
peeled and minced

½ teaspoon Ceylon cinnamon

½ teaspoon pure vanilla extract

1 tablespoon organic psyllium
husk

2 ice cubes

1 date, pitted, or 1 teaspoon raw
honey (optional)

OPTIONAL TOPPINGS

1 teaspoon buckwheat groats

1 tablespoon pomegranate
powder

½ sliced kiwi

3 blackberries

With turmeric, ginger, and cinnamon, this anti-inflammatory smoothie bowl is a body-detox bonanza! An ever-growing body of research shows that just a PINCH of turmeric may have a huge effect in reversing cellular damage. So drink up!

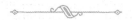

Place the coconut milk, banana, protein powder, almond butter, turmeric, ginger, cinnamon, vanilla, psyllium husk, ice cubes, and, if using, the date in a high-powered blender and puree until smooth. Dress with toppings, if desired.

MEAL MATH per serving			Toppings add 40 calories; 2g fiber			
calories	fat	sodium	carbs	fiber	sugar	protein
270	12g	115mg	37g	12g	13g	15g

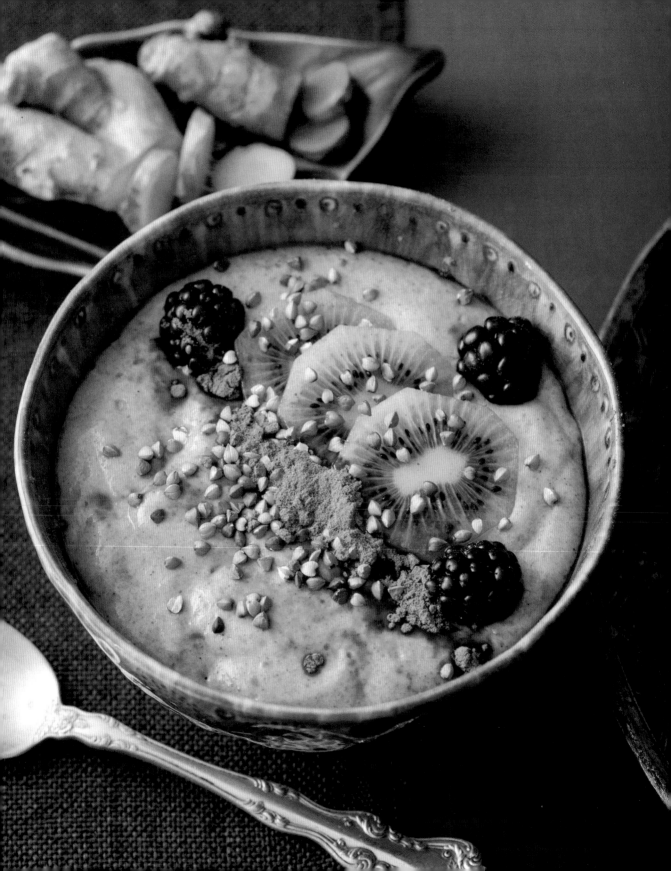

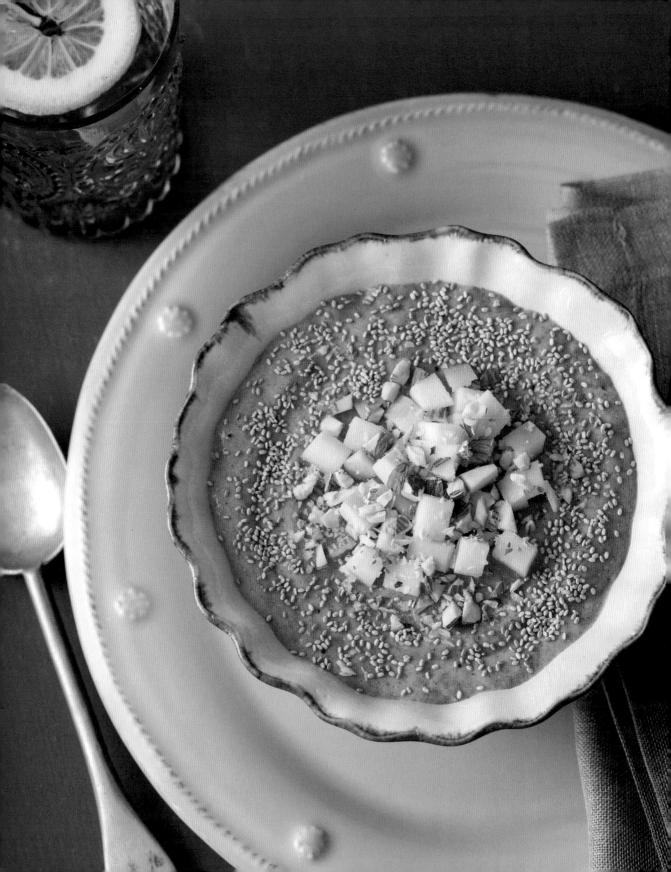

Apple-Teeny:
APPLE STRAWBERRY

MAKES 1 SERVING

V Vegan GF Gluten-free

Invite your friends over for an apple-teeny. Not as in the cocktail 'tini—I'm talking about something fun and delicious that packs a nutritional punch with over 150 percent of your recommended daily allowance of immune-boosting vitamin C! And with a megaload of fiber, this morning meal will keep your tummy satisfied and your waist teeny. Cheers!

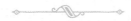

Place the milk, apple, almond butter, strawberries, psyllium husk, ice cubes, and, if using, the ginger in a high-powered blender and puree until smooth. Dress with toppings, if desired.

¾ cup unsweetened plant-based milk (see page 139)

1 small apple, peeled, cored, and roughly chopped

2 teaspoons almond butter or other nut butter

1 cup frozen strawberries

1 tablespoon psyllium husk or ground flaxseed

2 ice cubes

½-inch piece fresh ginger, peeled and minced (optional)

OPTIONAL TOPPINGS

2 teaspoons chia seeds

3 tablespoons diced apples

1 teaspoon sliced almonds

MEAL MATH per serving			Toppings add 63 calories; 4g fiber			
calories	fat	sodium	carbs	fiber	sugar	protein
220	8g	140mg	37g	14g	19g	4g

Happy Gut:
KEFIR POUR AND GO

MAKES 1 SERVING

 Gluten-free

1 cup organic plain 2% kefir

1 cup fresh or frozen raspberries

1 tablespoon chia seeds

2 teaspoons sliced almonds

1 teaspoon raw honey (optional)

OPTIONAL TOPPINGS

¼ teaspoon Ceylon cinnamon

¼ teaspoon granulated orange peel

The benefits of probiotics are bountiful—they help maintain a healthful balance of digestive flora. And kefir delivers a higher amount and a wider variety than regular yogurt! Your gut will be grateful when you whip up this juicy smoothie. Kefir also contains both calcium and vitamin D to keep your bones strong. Toss in some fiberlicious raspberries for a sweet, nutrient-loaded breakfast you can simply pour . . . and go!

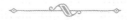

Pour the kefir and raspberries into a travel-size jar. Top with the chia seeds, almonds, and, if using, the raw honey. Dress with toppings, if desired.

MEAL MATH per serving						
calories	fat	sodium	carbs	fiber	sugar	protein
270	10g	210mg	28g	15g	17g	16g

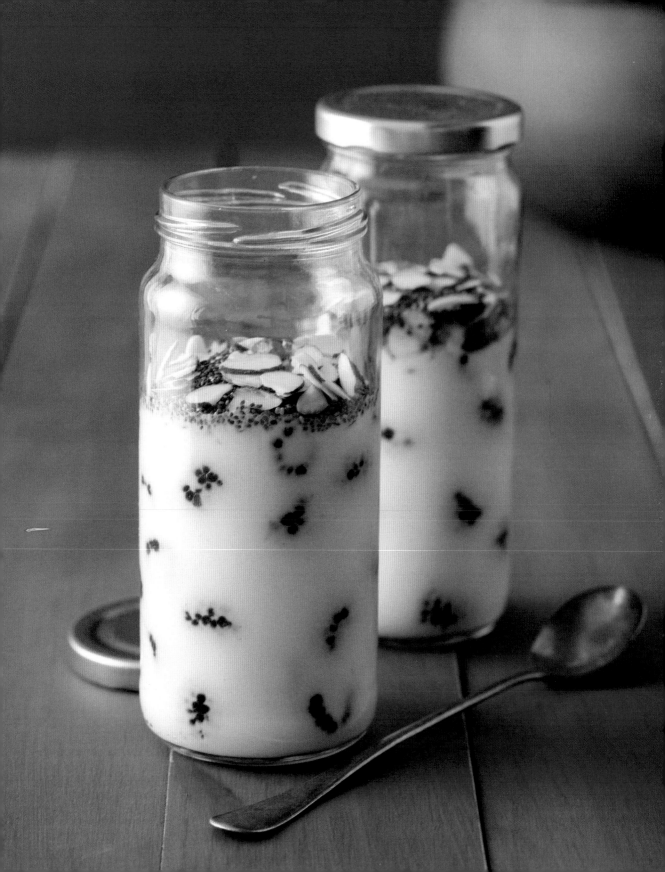

Do-It-Yourself:
ANATOMY OF A SMOOTHIE BOWL

ONCE YOU GET THE HANG OF SOUPING FOR BREAKFAST AND ARE IN THE MAINTENANCE PHASE OF THE PLAN, FEEL FREE TO MIX THINGS UP AND GET CREATIVE! JUST REFER TO MY BREAKFAST RULE OF 3 (SEE PAGES 158–159) AND YOU'RE GOOD TO BLEND AND GO.

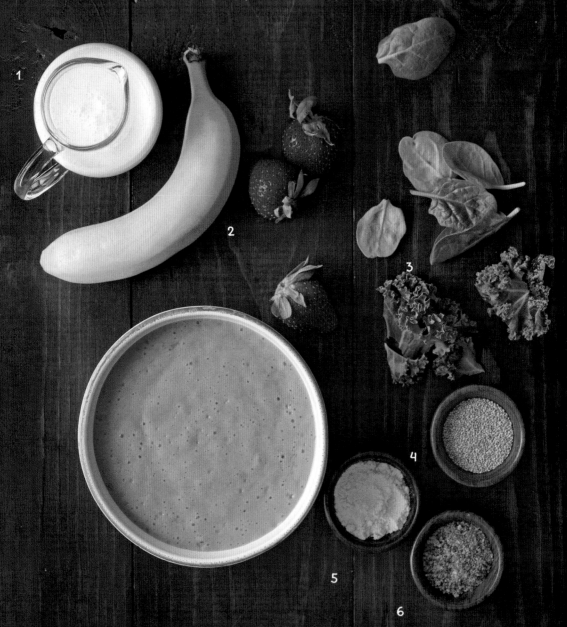

HERE'S MY SOUPER-BASIC SMOOTHIE BOWL FORMULA:

1. **LIQUID BASE: 1 CUP**
UNSWEETENED PLANT-BASED MILK (ALMOND, CASHEW, COCONUT, HEMP)
COCONUT WATER
FILTERED WATER

2. **FRUIT: 1 CUP**
1 SMALL BANANA
BERRIES
PEACH
MANGO
PINEAPPLE

3. **VEGETABLE: 1 CUP**
SPINACH
KALE

4. **FIBER BOOST: 1 TABLESPOON**
CHIA SEEDS
FLAXSEEDS
PSYLLIUM HUSK

5. **PROTEIN PUNCH**
1 TABLESPOON PLANT-BASED PROTEIN POWDER
1 TABLESPOON HEMP SEEDS
1/2 CUP ORGANIC PLAIN 2% GREEK YOGURT
1/2 CUP ORGANIC PLAIN 2% KEFIR

6. **POWER UP**
ADD ANY OF THE TOPPERS AND POWERFOOD POWDERS
ON THE FOLLOWING PAGES.

WANT TO ADD A LITTLE SOMETHING EXTRA TO YOUR NAKED BREAKFAST SOUP?

LET'S PLAY DRESS-UP! THESE TASTY TOPPERS NOT ONLY AMP UP THE NUTRITIONAL VALUE OF YOUR BOWL, BUT THEY ALSO PROVIDE A SATISFYING CRUNCH. TOSS ON WHATEVER TOPPING YOUR HEART (OR TUMMY) DESIRES—JUST MAKE SURE TO MEASURE THEM OUT SO THAT YOUR SMOOTHIE BOWL DOESN'T TOPPLE OVER THE 350-CALORIE LIMIT!

TOPPINGS	PER TABLESPOON	PER TEASPOON
ALMONDS, SLICED	33 CALORIES	11 CALORIES
ALMOND BUTTER	96 CALORIES	32 CALORIES
SPICED BUCKWHEAT GRANOLA (PAGE 137)	40 CALORIES	13 CALORIES
BUCKWHEAT GROATS	40 CALORIES	13 CALORIES
RAW CACAO NIBS	43 CALORIES	14 CALORIES
CASHEWS, CHOPPED	45 CALORIES	15 CALORIES
CHIA SEEDS	59 CALORIES	20 CALORIES
UNSWEETENED COCONUT FLAKES	24 CALORIES	8 CALORIES
FLAXSEED (GROUND)	37 CALORIES	12 CALORIES
FLAXSEED (WHOLE)	56 CALORIES	19 CALORIES
DRIED GOJI BERRIES	33 CALORIES	11 CALORIES
DRIED GOLDEN BERRIES	27 CALORIES	9 CALORIES
HEMP SEEDS	55 CALORIES	18 CALORIES
MULBERRIES	30 CALORIES	10 CALORIES
OAT BRAN	35 CALORIES	12 CALORIES
PEANUT BUTTER (ORGANIC)	96 CALORIES	32 CALORIES
PECANS, CHOPPED	47 CALORIES	16 CALORIES
PEPITAS (PUMPKIN SEEDS)	42 CALORIES	14 CALORIES
PINE NUTS	57 CALORIES	19 CALORIES
PISTACHIOS (SHELLED)	43 CALORIES	14 CALORIES
RAISINS	27 CALORIES	9 CALORIES
ROLLED OATS	38 CALORIES	13 CALORIES
SUNFLOWER SEEDS	46 CALORIES	15 CALORIES
WALNUTS, CHOPPED	48 CALORIES	16 CALORIES
WHEAT BRAN	8 CALORIES	3 CALORIES
WHEAT GERM	26 CALORIES	9 CALORIES

Power Up:
BREAKFAST BOWL TOPPERS

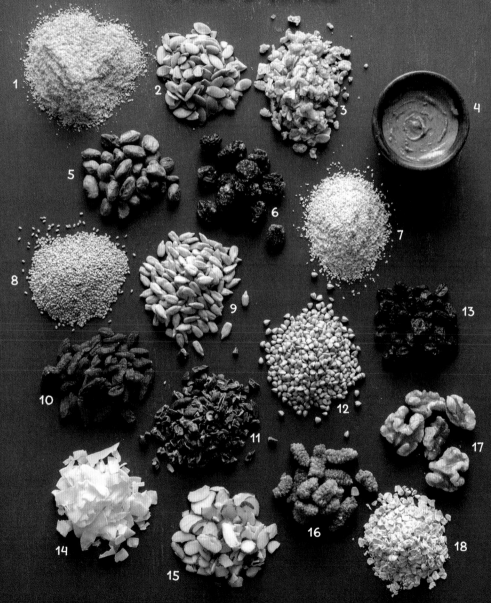

BREAKFAST BOWL TOPPERS: 1. WHEAT GERM; 2. PEPITAS; 3. GRANOLA; 4. ALMOND BUTTER;
5. PISTACHIOS; 6. DRIED GOLDEN BERRIES; 7. OAT BRAN; 8. WHITE CHIA SEEDS;
9. SUNFLOWER SEEDS; 10. DRIED GOJI BERRIES; 11. RAW CACAO NIBS; 12. BUCKWHEAT GROATS;
13. RAISINS; 14. UNSWEETENED COCONUT FLAKES; 15. ALMOND SLICES;
16. MULBERRIES; 17. WALNUTS; 18. ROLLED OATS

Power Up:
POWERFOOD POWDERS

AMPLIFY THE NUTRI-POWER OF YOUR MORNING MEAL WITH ANY OF THESE POWERFOOD POWDERS.

THEY HAVE ALL THE NUTRITION FROM WHOLE FOODS CRAMMED INTO A FINE POWDER, SO JUST A SMALL SPOONFUL GIVES YOUR BREAKFAST A MAJOR UPGRADE WITH SERIOUS ANTIOXIDIZING AND BODY-HEALING BENEFITS. IN A NUTSHELL, YOU'RE ADDING A LOT MORE GOOD TO YOUR A.M. MEAL.

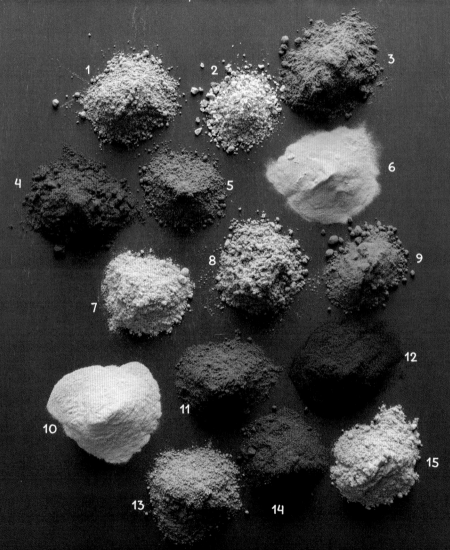

POWERFOOD POWDERS: 1. BROCCOLI SPROUT; 2. ORANGE PEEL; 3. ACAI;
4. RASPBERRY; 5. CACAO; 6. POMEGRANATE; 7. PRICKLY PEAR; 8. KALE;
9. TURMERIC; 10. PUMPKIN; 11. CINNAMON; 12. BEET;
13. MATCHA; 14. BLACKBERRY; 15. GINGER

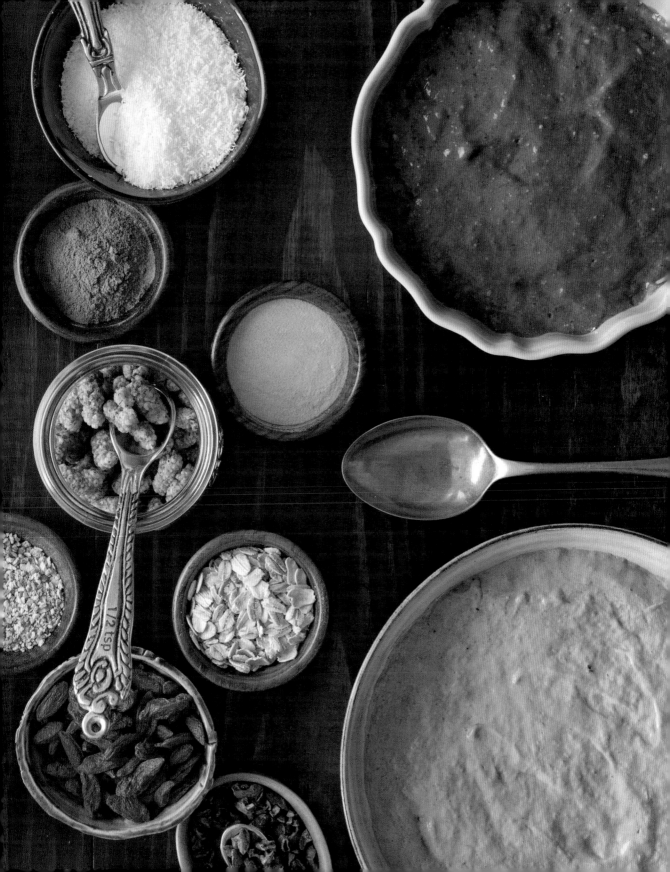

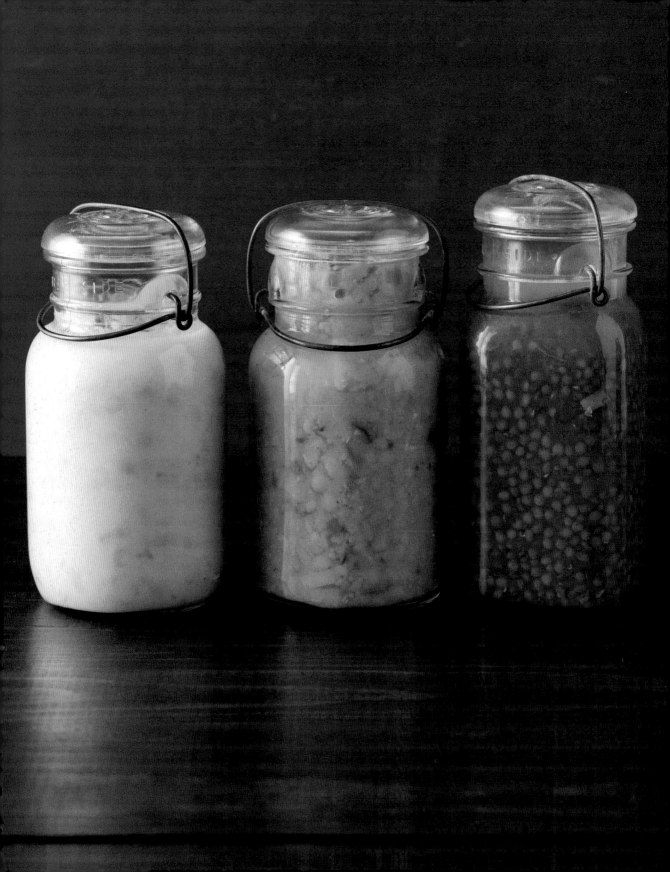

Lunch and Dinner

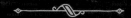

Detox without deprivation! All of these soups have been carefully designed so that every bowl is a complete meal—I've done the math to ensure you get the right balance of filling protein, fiber, and healthful fat, plus tons of cell-protecting antioxidants, all with a caloric content that'll make the pounds fall off. There's something for everyone: comfort soups, traditional recipes, exotic flavors, as well as soups that are vegan and gluten-free.

Happy souping!

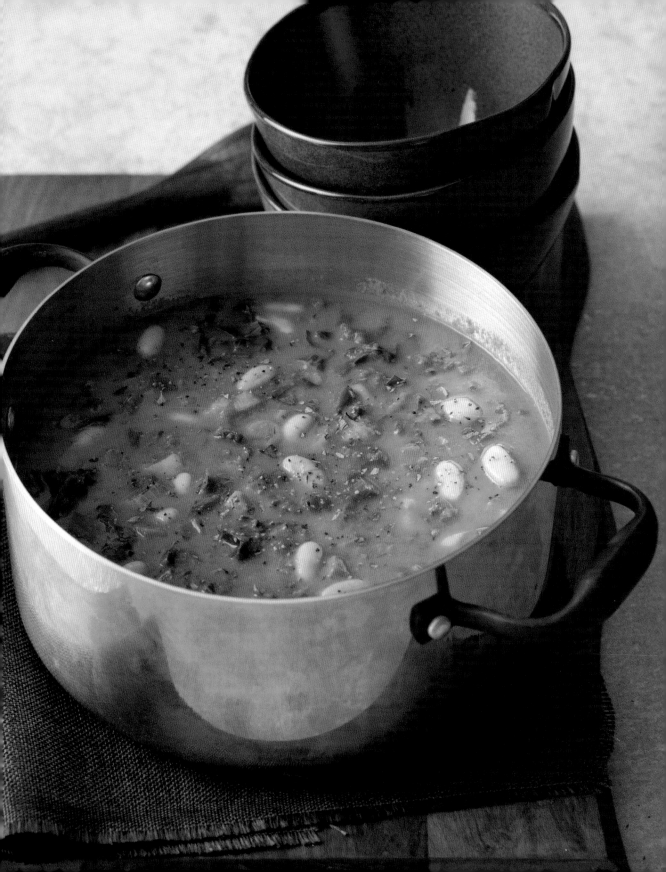

Ignite Me:
TUSCAN-STYLE WHITE BEAN

MAKES 4 SERVINGS (SERVING SIZE: 2 CUPS)

V *Vegan*   **GF** *Gluten-free*

This is one of my fiery faves, kissing your lips and igniting your tongue with red pepper flakes—which, by the way, contain capsaicin, a powerful inflammation fighter that may help burn body fat and combat cardiovascular disease. So protect your heart while making others' pound at the sight of you.

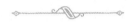

Heat the oil in a large pot over medium heat. Add the onion, garlic, carrots, and celery and sauté 5 minutes, until softened. Stir in the tomato paste and allow it to caramelize on the bottom of the pot, about 3 minutes more. Add the tomatoes and broth and bring the soup to a boil. Reduce the heat and simmer, covered, for 15 minutes, until the veggies are cooked through. Carefully place half of the soup in a high-powered blender and puree until smooth, then pour it back into the pot. Add the Swiss chard, beans, oregano, and red pepper flakes and simmer for 6 to 8 minutes, until tender. Season with salt and pepper to taste and serve.

1 tablespoon extra-virgin olive oil

1 medium onion, chopped

3 cloves garlic, minced

2 medium carrots, chopped

3 stalks celery, chopped

2 tablespoons tomato paste

2 large tomatoes, chopped

4 cups low-sodium vegetable broth

Bunch of Swiss chard, chopped (about 6 cups)

3 cups cooked cannellini beans, no salt added

2 tablespoons minced fresh oregano

½ teaspoon red pepper flakes

Himalayan or sea salt and freshly ground black pepper

Power Up!

ADD TO YOUR POT:

½ teaspoon ground cayenne pepper, with the other spices

1 tablespoon chopped jalapeño, for finishing

ADD TO YOUR BOWL:

1 tablespoon Powerfood Pesto (page 204) or 1 tablespoon nut of your choice

MEAL MATH per serving						
calories	*fat*	*sodium*	*carbs*	*fiber*	*sugar*	*protein*
280	6g	420mg	46g	14g	10g	13g

loat Me:

↓ PEA, ASPARAGUS,
⌐ᵣₐₛₗₑᵧ PARSLEY

MAKES 6 SERVINGS (SERVING SIZE: 2 CUPS)

V Vegan   **GF** Gluten-free

1 tablespoon coconut oil

1½ cups chopped leeks

8 cups low-sodium
vegetable broth

6 cups frozen green peas

2 bunches of asparagus (30 to
40 stalks), tough ends removed
and cut into 1-inch pieces

½ cup chopped fresh parsley

Himalayan or sea salt and
freshly ground black pepper

Power Up!

ADD TO YOUR POT:

2 teaspoons minced fresh
thyme (stir in with the parsley)

ADD TO YOUR BOWL:

1 tablespoon Cashew Crème
(page 206) or Sesame Kale Pesto
(page 203)

A Hollywood favorite during award season among my celebrity clients, this tummy debloater is my delicious red-carpet-ready trick of the trade. The secret in this soup is the parsley, which helps flush out excess water from the body and keeps tummy bloat at bay. Plus, asparagus is rich in vitamins A, E, C, and K, and the green peas are high in protein and loaded with all types of B vitamins that may help energize you. I think of this trio of powergreens as a tasty multivitamin in a bowl!

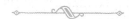

Heat the oil in a large pot over medium heat. Add the leeks and sauté for 4 minutes, until softened. Add the broth and bring to a simmer. Stir in the peas and asparagus and simmer, covered, for 3 minutes longer. Carefully place half of the soup in a high-powered blender and puree until smooth, then return it to the pot. Add the parsley and stir well to combine. Season with salt and pepper to taste and serve.

MEAL MATH per serving						
calories	fat	sodium	carbs	fiber	sugar	protein
210	3g	200mg	36g	12g	13g	13g

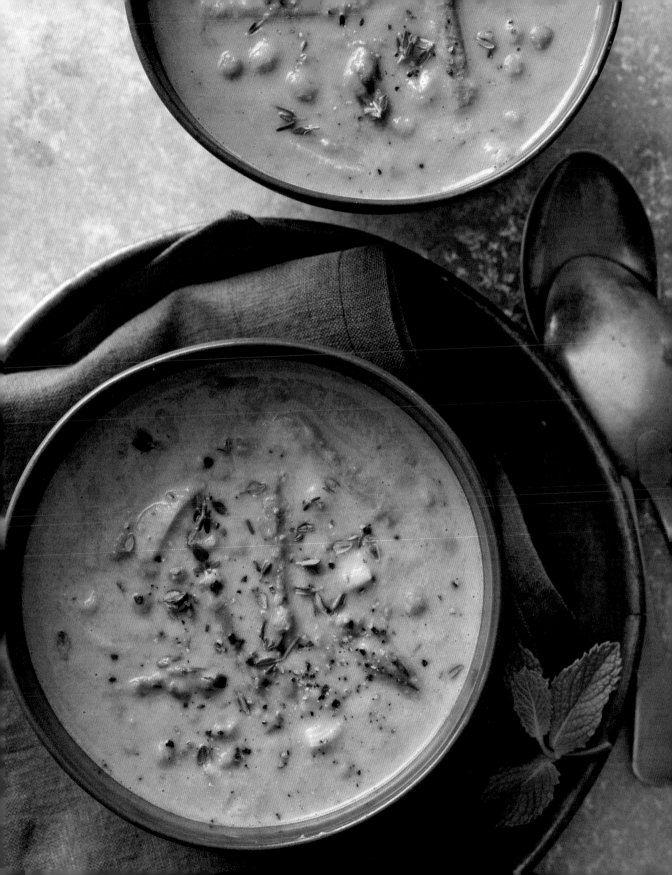

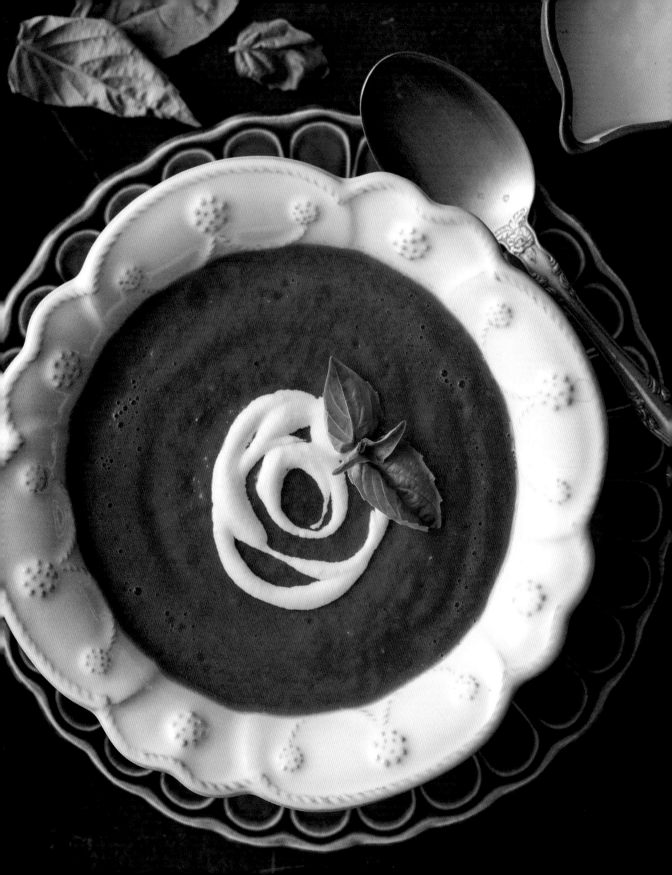

Comfort Me:
CREAMY TOMATO

MAKES 4 SERVINGS (SERVING SIZE: 2 CUPS)

V *Vegan*   **GF** *Gluten-free*

Who doesn't crave a nice cup of creamy soup? Just thinking about it makes you feel warm and comfy,. This soup is velvety and lush thanks to a surprise ingredient: cannellini beans. They're a brilliant stand-in for heavy cream—giving the dish a similar full-bodied flavor, minus the gazillions of extra calories. And with 12 grams of fiber per serving, this soup is seriously satisfying.

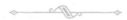

Heat the oil in a large pot over medium heat. Add the onion and sauté 3 to 5 minutes, until softened. Add the tomatoes, beans, and broth and simmer, covered, for 20 minutes. Uncover and simmer for 10 minutes more, stirring occasionally. Add the basil. Carefully pour the soup into a high-powered blender and puree until smooth. Season with salt and pepper to taste and serve.

1 tablespoon extra-virgin olive oil

1 medium onion, chopped

12 Roma tomatoes, chopped

3 cups cooked cannellini beans, no salt added

2 cups low-sodium vegetable broth

8 fresh basil leaves

Himalayan or sea salt and freshly ground black pepper

Power Up!

ADD TO YOUR BOWL:

1½ tablespoons Cashew Crème (page 206)

Fresh basil leaves

MEAL MATH *per serving*						
calories	*fat*	*sodium*	*carbs*	*fiber*	*sugar*	*protein*
250	5g	150mg	41g	12g	11g	12g

Sustain Me:
VEG-LOADED LENTIL

MAKES 6 SERVINGS (SERVING SIZE: 2 CUPS)

V Vegan **GF** Gluten-free

1 tablespoon extra-virgin olive oil or avocado oil

1 medium onion, chopped

1 medium carrot, chopped

2 stalks celery, chopped

2 cups dried French green lentils

1 large tomato, chopped

8 cups filtered water

2 medium zucchini, chopped

4 cups baby spinach

2 cloves garlic, minced

Himalayan or sea salt and freshly ground black pepper

Power Up!

ADD TO YOUR POT:

½ teaspoon ground turmeric and/or 1 teaspoon ground cumin (along with zucchini)

1 tablespoon minced fresh rosemary (for finishing)

ADD TO YOUR BOWL:

1 tablespoon hemp seeds

Every other week I make a big batch of this for my team. It keeps everyone full, energized, and satisfied. Not only is this lentil-and-veggie soup delicious, but it's also a cinch to make, lasts for days in the fridge, and is a hit with the entire family (home and office). Leftovers you can get excited about? Sign me up!

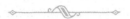

Heat the oil in a large pot over medium heat. Add the onion, carrot, and celery and sauté for 3 to 5 minutes, until softened. Stir in the lentils and tomato and cook for another 2 minutes. Add the water and bring the soup to a boil. Reduce the heat, cover, and simmer for 20 minutes, then stir in the zucchini, spinach, and garlic. Season with salt and pepper to taste and serve.

MEAL MATH per serving						
calories	fat	sodium	carbs	fiber	sugar	protein
280	3.5g	65mg	47g	9g	4g	18g

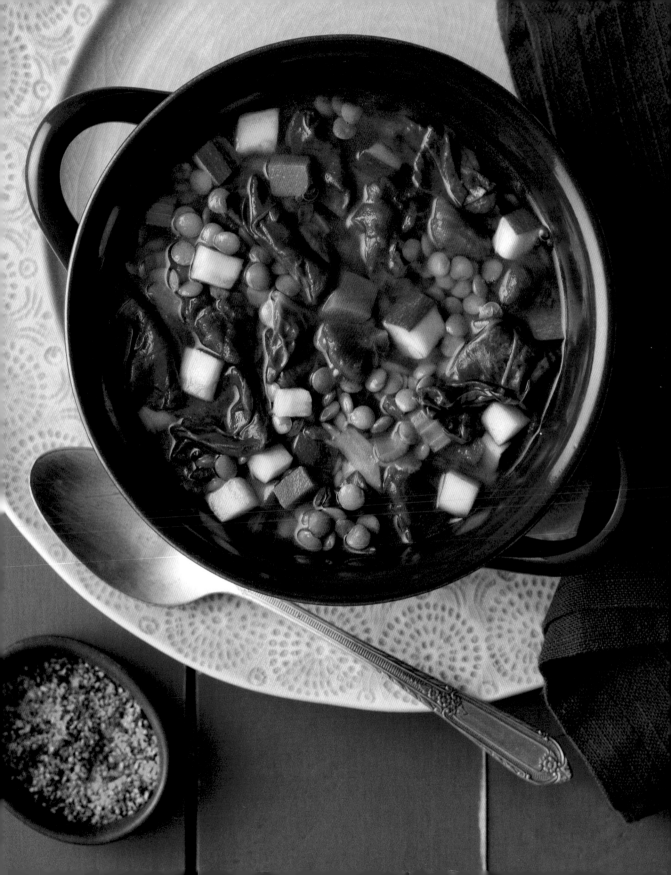

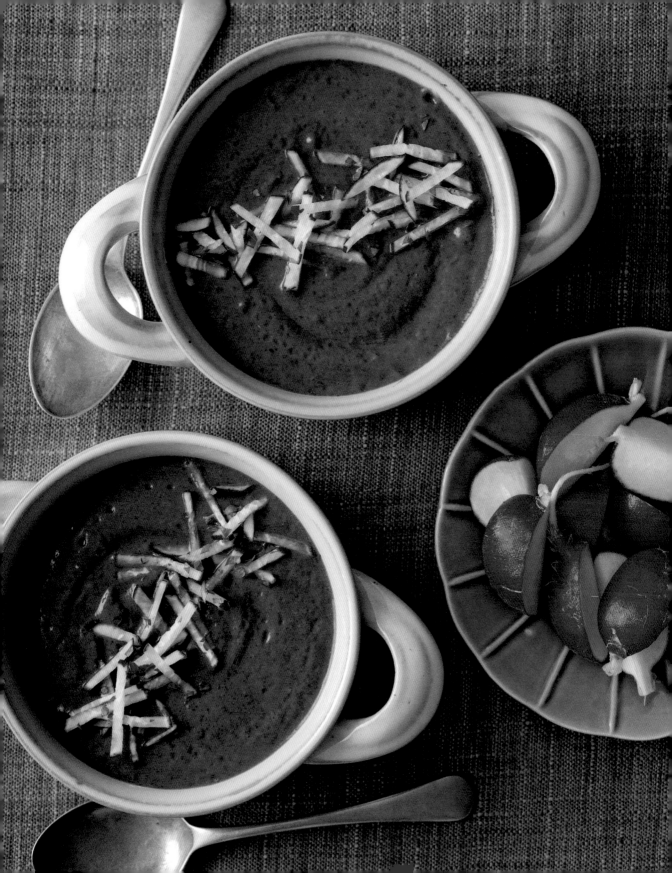

Fired Up:
SMOKY BLACK BEAN

MAKES 4 SERVINGS (SERVING SIZE: 2 CUPS)

V *Vegan*   **GF** *Gluten-free*

The name doesn't lie—this flavorful soup is smoky, spicy, and completely satisfying thanks to the fiber- and protein-rich black beans. In addition, the red pepper flakes give this soup a kick that studies have shown may rev up metabolism and help you burn more body fat. Top it off with extra herbs or some sliced avocado for additional flavor and healthful fat. Can't argue with that!

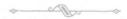

Heat the oil in a large pot over medium heat. Add the onion and garlic and sauté for 3 to 5 minutes, until softened. Add the beans, red pepper flakes, cumin, thyme, cauliflower, and broth and bring to a boil. Reduce the heat and simmer, covered, for 10 to 15 minutes, until the veggies are tender. Carefully pour the soup into a high-powered blender and puree until smooth. Season with salt and pepper to taste and serve.

1 tablespoon extra-virgin olive oil

1 medium onion, chopped

3 cloves garlic, minced

3 cups cooked black beans, no salt added

¼ teaspoon red pepper flakes

1 tablespoon ground cumin

1 teaspoon minced fresh thyme

Medium head of cauliflower, chopped

6 cups low-sodium vegetable broth

Himalayan or sea salt and freshly ground black pepper

Power Up!

ADD TO YOUR BOWL:

1 to 2 tablespoons minced fresh herb of your choice

¼ avocado, diced

MEAL MATH per serving						
calories	fat	sodium	carbs	fiber	sugar	protein
280	6g	260mg	44g	15g	6g	16g

Squash Soirée:
GARDEN-GREEN MINESTRONE

MAKES 6 SERVINGS (SERVING SIZE 2½ CUPS)

V Vegan　　GF Gluten-free

1 tablespoon extra-virgin olive oil

1 medium onion, chopped

2 cloves garlic, minced

2 medium yellow squash, chopped

2 medium zucchini, chopped

1 medium carrot, chopped

3 large tomatoes, chopped

8 cups low-sodium vegetable broth

3 cups cooked kidney beans, no salt added

2 cups baby spinach

2 cups chopped kale

Himalayan or sea salt and freshly ground black pepper

Things get a whole lot healthier when you invite chopped squash and fresh leafy greens to your minestrone bowl. Everything about this soup shouts SPRING! And with its abundance of fiber and antioxidant-rich kidney beans along with an extra boost of veg, this soup will give your party a delicious nutritional edge.

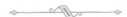

Heat the oil in a large pot over medium heat. Add the onion and sauté 3 to 5 minutes, until softened. Add the garlic and cook 1 more minute. Stir in the squash, zucchini, and carrot and sauté for 5 minutes. Add the tomatoes and broth and bring to a boil. Reduce the heat and simmer, covered, for 20 minutes. Add the beans, spinach, and kale and simmer for another 10 minutes, stirring occasionally. Season with salt and pepper to taste and serve.

Power Up!

ADD TO YOUR POT:

1 teaspoon ground cumin or ½ teaspoon red pepper flakes (along with tomatoes)

ADD TO YOUR BOWL:

1 tablespoon pine nuts or pepitas, or 2 teaspoons chili oil

MEAL MATH per serving						
calories	fat	sodium	carbs	fiber	sugar	protein
320	3g	280mg	39g	17g	6g	15g

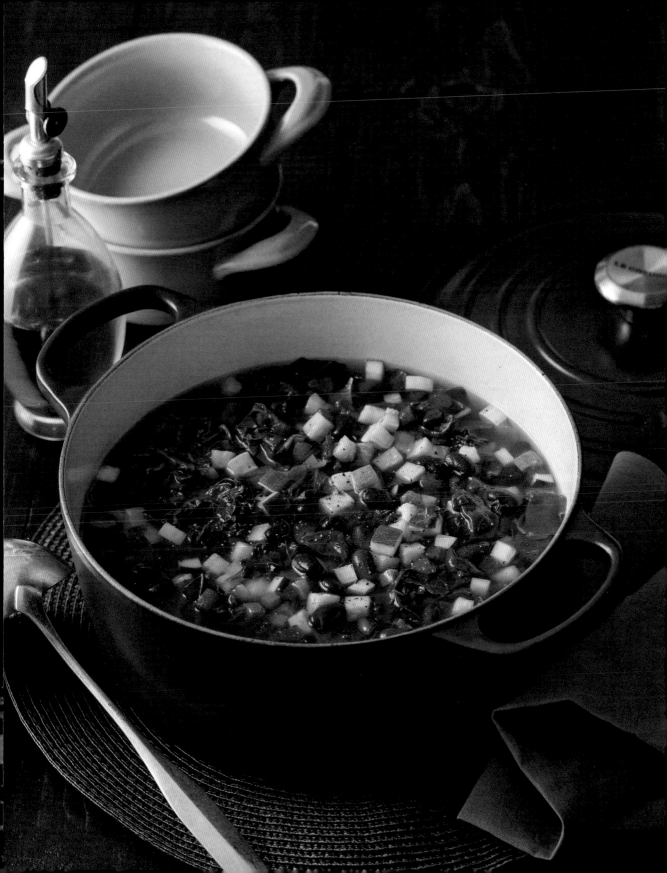

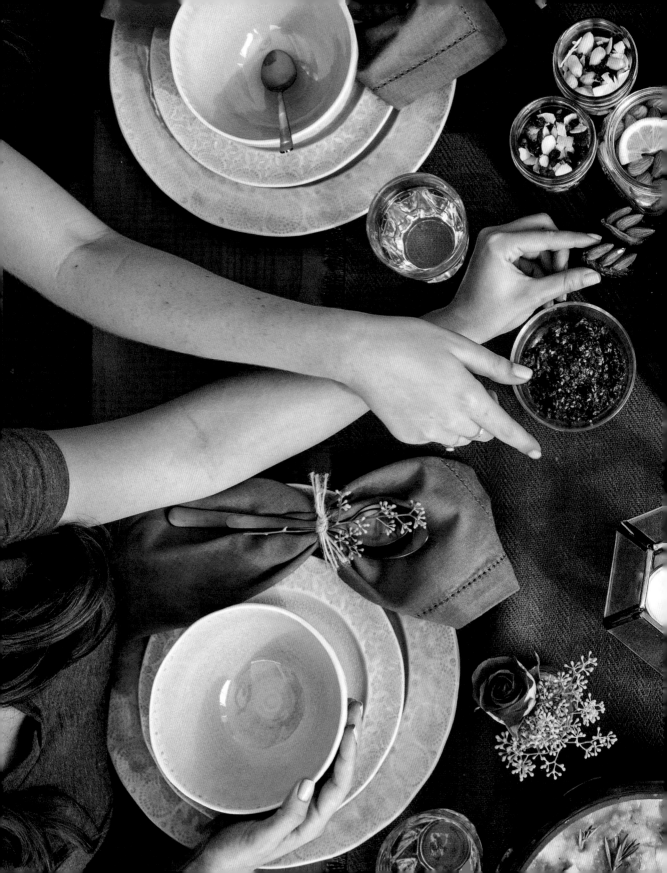

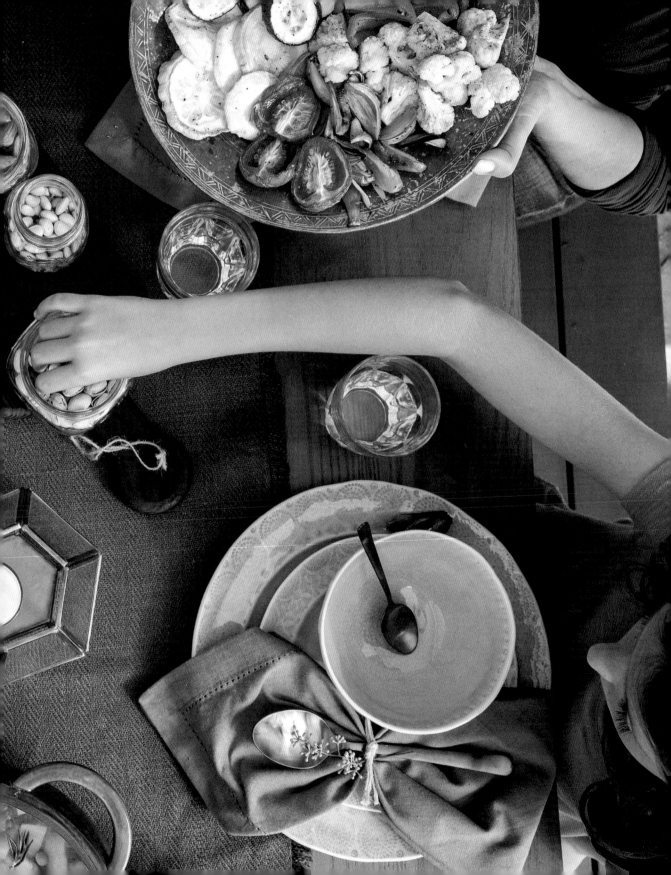

Warm Me: RED LENTIL

MAKES 4 SERVINGS (SERVING SIZE: 2 CUPS)

V Vegan   **GF** Gluten-free

2 tablespoons extra-virgin olive oil or coconut oil

1 medium onion, chopped

1½ cups dried red lentils

1 teaspoon garlic powder

1 medium carrot, chopped

½ cup tomato puree

8 cups filtered water or low-sodium vegetable broth

4 tablespoons minced fresh cilantro or 2 tablespoons dried

Himalayan or sea salt and freshly ground black pepper

Power Up!

ADD TO YOUR BOWL:

1 to 2 tablespoons minced fresh cilantro

¼ teaspoon red pepper flakes

If you've never tried red lentils before, I encourage you to give them a taste test. Their mildly sweet and nutty flavor sets them apart from the traditional brown ones, and the cilantro gives this comforting soup an exotic appeal. Cool fact: This herb is a good source of iron and magnesium, which may help fight anemia. It could also help relieve gas (see ya, bloat!) and aid in digestion (sayonara, belly bulge!). Sprinkle extra cilantro on top of the dish for detox bonus points.

———— ❧ ————

Heat the oil in a large pot over medium heat. Add the onion and sauté 3 to 5 minutes, until softened. Add the lentils, garlic powder, carrot, tomato puree, water, and cilantro and bring to a boil. Reduce the heat to low and cook, covered, for 30 to 45 minutes, until the lentils are tender. Season with salt and pepper to taste and serve with a side of veg.

MEAL MATH per serving						
calories	fat	sodium	carbs	fiber	sugar	protein
260	7g	55mg	36g	15g	4g	13g

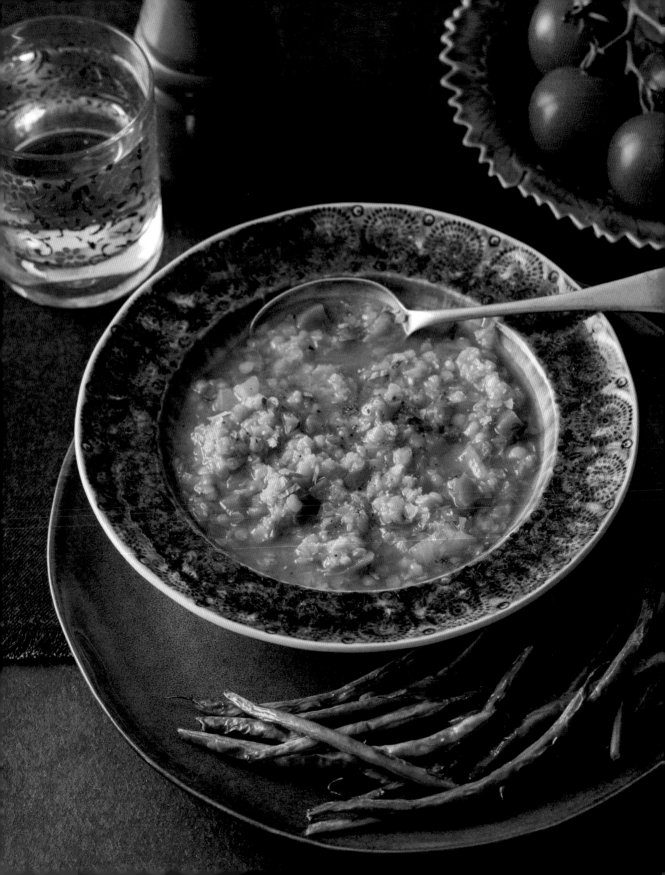

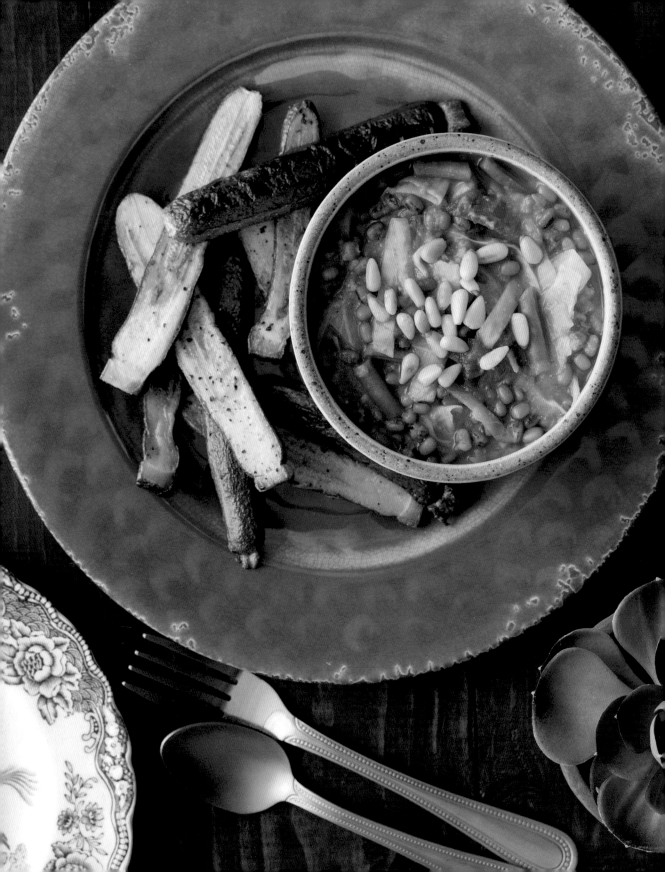

Zen-Sational: MUNG BEAN

MAKES 8 SERVINGS (SERVING SIZE: 2 CUPS)

V Vegan   **GF** Gluten-free

What are mung beans? They're kind of like lentils: quick-cooking with a flavorful, nutty taste. But don't let their delicate flavor mask their mighty-mung health potentials—these babies are full of all-important protein, fiber, and folate. Plus, they're packed with phyto-chemicals that may help protect your cells from damage. Enlighten your taste buds with every spoonful.

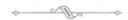

Heat the oil in a large pot over medium heat. Add the onion and sauté 3 to 5 minutes, until softened. Add the mung beans and sauté for an additional 2 minutes. Add the celery, green beans, and carrot and sauté for 3 to 5 minutes. Add the broth, bring to a boil, and simmer for about 45 minutes. Stir in the cabbage and tomatoes and simmer for an additional 10 minutes. The cabbage should remain crunchy. Season with salt and pepper to taste and serve.

1 tablespoon extra-virgin olive oil

1 medium onion, chopped

2½ cups dried mung beans, rinsed

2 stalks celery, chopped

2 cups green beans, chopped

1 medium carrot, chopped

12 cups low-sodium vegetable broth

4 cups thinly sliced green cabbage

2 medium tomatoes, chopped

Himalayan or sea salt and freshly ground black pepper

Power Up!

ADD TO YOUR BOWL:

1 tablespoon pine nuts

¼ teaspoon red pepper flakes

MEAL MATH *per serving*						
calories	*fat*	*sodium*	*carbs*	*fiber*	*sugar*	*protein*
260	3g	420mg	44g	13g	7g	16g

Strengthen Me:
SAVORY SPLIT PEA

MAKES 6 SERVINGS (SERVING SIZE: 1½ CUPS)

V *Vegan*   **GF** *Gluten-free*

1 tablespoon extra-virgin olive oil

1 medium onion, chopped

2 medium carrots, chopped

2 stalks celery, chopped

2 cups dried split green peas, rinsed

8 cups filtered water

Himalayan or sea salt and freshly ground black pepper

Power Up!

ADD TO YOUR BOWL:

1 tablespoon Cashew Crème (page 206)

Peas are sneaky little greens—sure, they may camouflage themselves as vegetables, but each serving of this soup actually provides 17 grams of protein! As if that weren't devious enough, these sophisticated little guys add hefty amounts of vitamins A, K, and of course fiber to this simple, filling soup. So when it's midafternoon and hunger strikes, all we are saying is give peas a chance. To make it a complete meal, serve with a side of roasted broccoli or kale, adding extra crunch and cruciferous power.

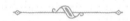

Heat the oil in a large pot over medium heat. Add the onion and sauté 3 to 5 minutes, until softened. Add carrots and celery and sauté for another 2 to 3 minutes. Stir in the split peas and water and bring to a boil. Reduce the heat, cover, and simmer for 60 minutes, stirring occasionally until peas are cooked through and soft. Season with salt and pepper to taste. Serve with a side of veg.

Optional: For a super-smooth consistency, puree in a high-powered blender.

MEAL MATH per serving						
calories	fat	sodium	carbs	fiber	sugar	protein
290	3.5g	270mg	49g	18g	8g	17g

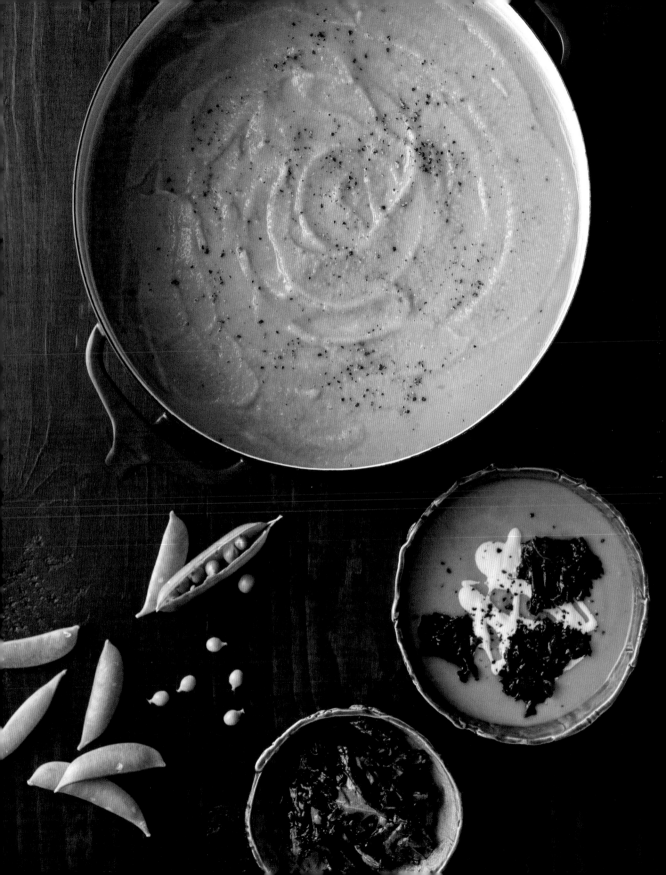

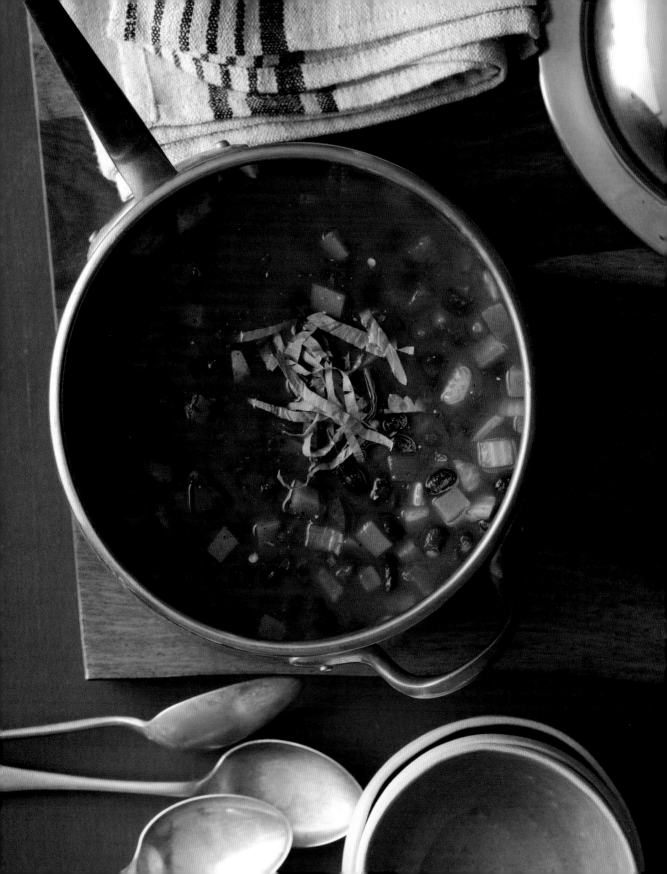

Fulfill Me:
HEARTY BLACK BEAN

MAKES 4 SERVINGS (SERVING SIZE: 2 CUPS)

V Vegan   **GF** Gluten-free

Beans, beans, the magical fruits, the more you eat, the cuter your glutes. These muscle-building bad boys deliver fiber, folate, and potential cancer-fighting saponins that have been shown to protect our cells and nourish our bodies. With more than thirty different kinds of antioxidants, this chunky meal is hearty, delicious, and most of all, fulfilling! Grab your spoon and slurp your way to powerfood satisfaction. Top it off with one of my suggested Power Ups and your meal is complete.

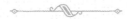

Heat the oil in a large pot over medium heat. Add the onion and sauté for 3 to 5 minutes. Stir in the carrots and bell pepper and sauté 2 minutes longer. Add the tomato puree, broth, and beans and bring to a boil. Reduce the heat, cover, and simmer for 30 minutes. Turn off the heat, stir in the garlic, red pepper flakes, and salt and pepper to taste; let stand, covered, for 10 minutes, then serve.

1 tablespoon extra-virgin olive oil

1 medium onion, chopped

2 medium carrots, chopped

1 medium red bell pepper, cored, seeded, and diced

1 cup tomato puree

4 cups low-sodium vegetable broth

3 cups cooked black beans, no salt added

3 cloves garlic, minced

¼ teaspoon red pepper flakes

Himalayan or sea salt and freshly ground black pepper

Power Up!

ADD TO YOUR BOWL:

¼ avocado or 1 tablespoon pepitas

Handful of chopped fresh cilantro or green onions

MEAL MATH per serving							
calories	fat	sodium	carbs	fiber	sugar	protein
270	5g	190mg	43g	13g	8g	13g

Nurture Me:
MAMA BELLER'S CHICKEN SOUP

MAKES 6 SERVINGS (SERVING SIZE: 2 CUPS)

GF *Gluten-free*

10 cups low-sodium chicken broth

5 cloves garlic

1 medium onion

1 parsnip, chopped in half

3 large skinless, bone-in organic chicken breasts

3 large carrots, cut into big chunks

2 stalks celery, cut into big chunks

3 medium zucchini, cut into big chunks

2 large yellow squash, cut into big chunks

Bunch of fresh parsley

Himalayan or sea salt

Power Up!

ADD TO YOUR BOWL:

Chopped celery leaves

Mama Beller (that's me) strongly recommends this soup when you've got a case of the sniffles. And it's not just an old wives' tale (tip: don't call me an old wife ☺). Science supports the idea that chicken soup can actually help you get over a cold—perhaps through the synergistic action of the veg and chicken. Ditch the can—this version, passed down from my own mama, is low in calories and sodium but top notch in health-boosting veg!

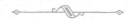

Pour the broth into a large pot and bring to a boil. Add the garlic, onion, parsnip, and chicken, reduce the heat and simmer, covered, for 1 hour. Remove the chicken and place in a large bowl to cool, then shred it with your fingers. Discard the bones and set aside. Add the carrots, celery, zucchini, squash, and parsley to the pot and continue to simmer for 30 minutes, leaving the lid slightly open, until vegetables soften. Season with salt to taste. Divide the shredded chicken among six bowls, ladle the soup on top, and serve.

MEAL MATH per serving						
calories	fat	sodium	carbs	fiber	sugar	protein
260	4.5g	310mg	21g	5g	11g	33g

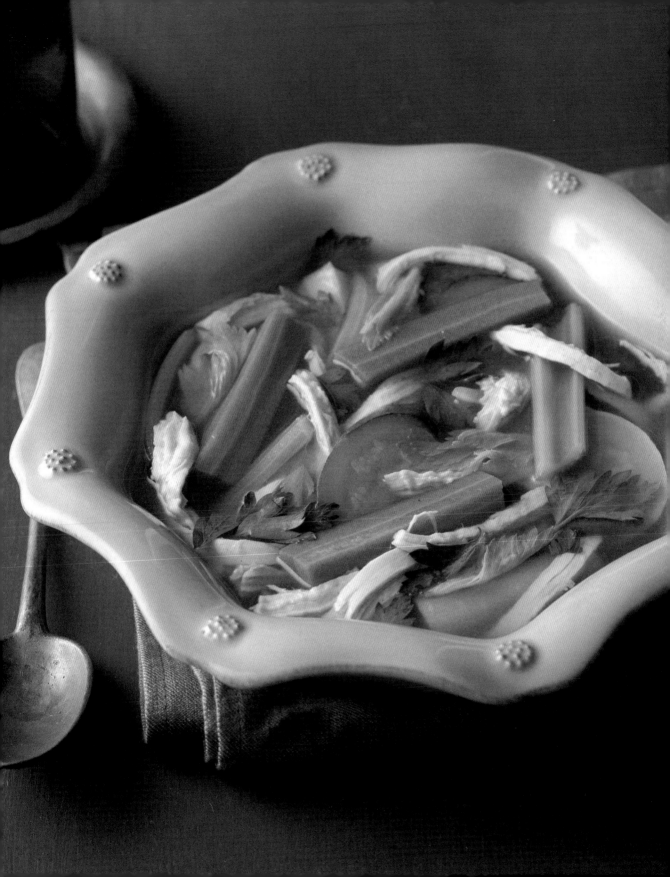

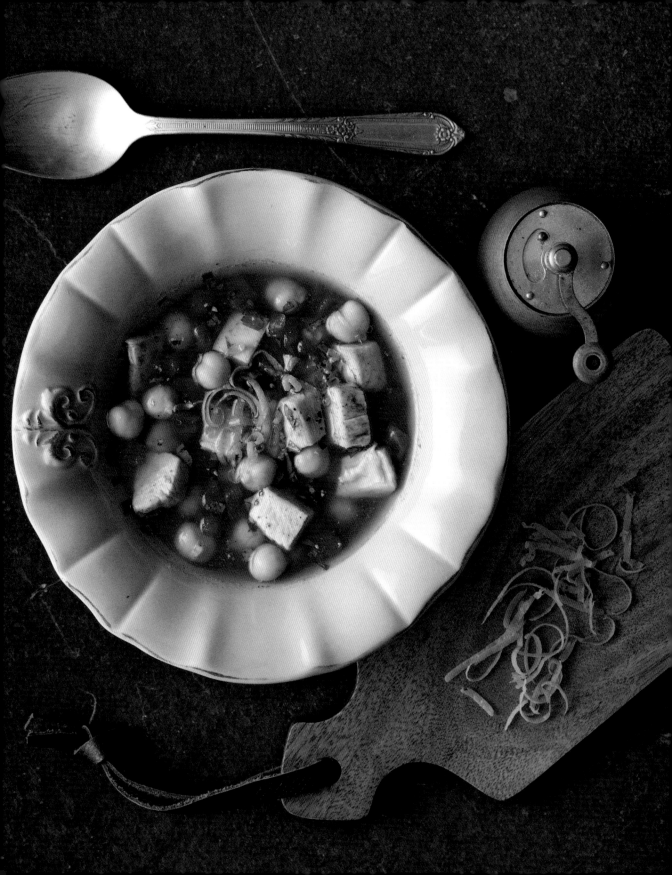

Souper Zesty:
ORANGE CHICKEN DONE RIGHT

MAKES 4 SERVINGS (SERVING SIZE: 2 CUPS)

GF *Gluten-free*

Ever order orange chicken from a Chinese restaurant? Sure, it tastes great—but it's essentially an orange-flavored fried donut stuffed with chicken fat, that's what. Mmmmm.

Here's an amazing alternative: fresh orange zest and aromatic spices make this dish taste like orange chicken but minus the fried coating, food coloring, sugar, and salt! And there's a ton of nutrition in that peel, too. Research shows that just a tiny amount contains limonene and hesperidin—code for heart-healthful compounds that may even help to suppress your appetite. Go ahead and play chicken—the right way.

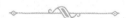

Heat the oil in a large pot over medium heat. Add the onion and garlic and sauté for 3 to 5 minutes, until softened. Stir in the chicken, cumin, and coriander. Add the orange zest and juice, chickpeas, tomatoes, and broth and bring to a boil. Reduce the heat and simmer, covered, for 20 minutes, until the chicken is cooked through. Add the lemon juice, season with salt and pepper to taste, and serve with a side of veg.

1 tablespoon extra-virgin olive oil

1 medium onion, chopped

2 cloves garlic, minced

2 skinless, boneless organic chicken breasts, cut into bite-size pieces

3 teaspoons ground cumin

3 teaspoons ground coriander

Zest and juice of 1 orange

1½ cups cooked chickpeas, no salt added

1½ cups diced tomatoes, no salt added

4 cups low-sodium vegetable broth

2 tablespoons freshly squeezed lemon juice

Himalayan or sea salt and freshly ground black pepper

Power Up!

ADD TO YOUR POT:

¼ cup chopped fresh parsley (along with the lemon juice)

ADD TO YOUR BOWL:

1 tablespoon orange zest

MEAL MATH per serving						
calories	fat	sodium	carbs	fiber	sugar	protein
340	8g	240mg	32g	8g	8g	35g

Greeeeen 5:
GREENS, BEANS, AND THINGS

MAKES 4 SERVINGS (SERVING SIZE: 2 CUPS)

V Vegan   **GF** Gluten-free

2 tablespoons extra-virgin olive oil

2 leeks, chopped

3 cloves garlic, sliced

Bunch of asparagus (15 to 20 stalks), tough ends removed, and cut into 1-inch pieces, or 3 cups chopped broccoli florets

2 cups frozen green peas

3 tablespoons chopped fresh parsley

6 cups low-sodium vegetable broth

1½ cups cooked cannellini beans, no salt added

Himalayan or sea salt

2 cups baby spinach

Freshly ground black pepper

Power Up!

ADD TO YOUR BOWL:

1 tablespoon hemp seeds

¼ cup chopped watercress

This tasteful twist on classic veggie soup is overflowing with good-for-you greens. Asparagus has more glutathione—one of our body's most powerful antioxidants—than any other fruit or vegetable that's been analyzed. It's a health superstar in my book! Coupled with inflammation-fighting leeks, this flavorful and cleansing bowl has got your back.

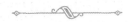

Heat the oil in a large pot over medium heat. Add the leeks and sauté until tender, about 5 minutes. Add the garlic and sauté another 2 minutes. Stir in the asparagus, peas, and parsley, then pour in the broth and beans and sprinkle with salt. Bring the soup to a boil, then reduce the heat and simmer, uncovered, until the veggies are just tender, 3 to 4 minutes. Stir in the spinach leaves, add salt and pepper to taste, and serve.

Variation: This soup also tastes great pureed—my favorite way to enjoy this soup is to puree half of the pot in a high-powered blender.

MEAL MATH per serving						
calories	fat	sodium	carbs	fiber	sugar	protein
280	8g	340mg	41g	12g	10g	14g

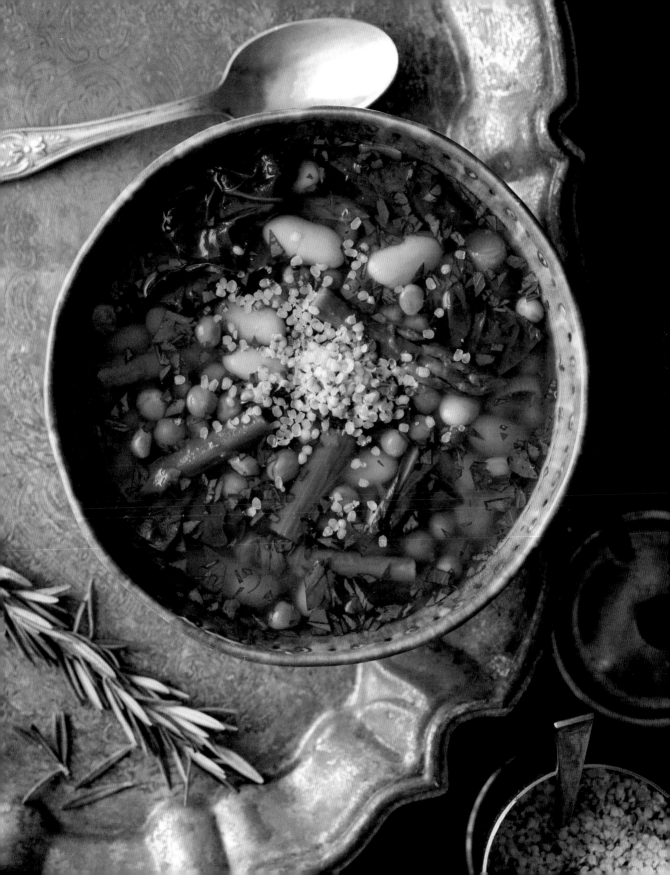

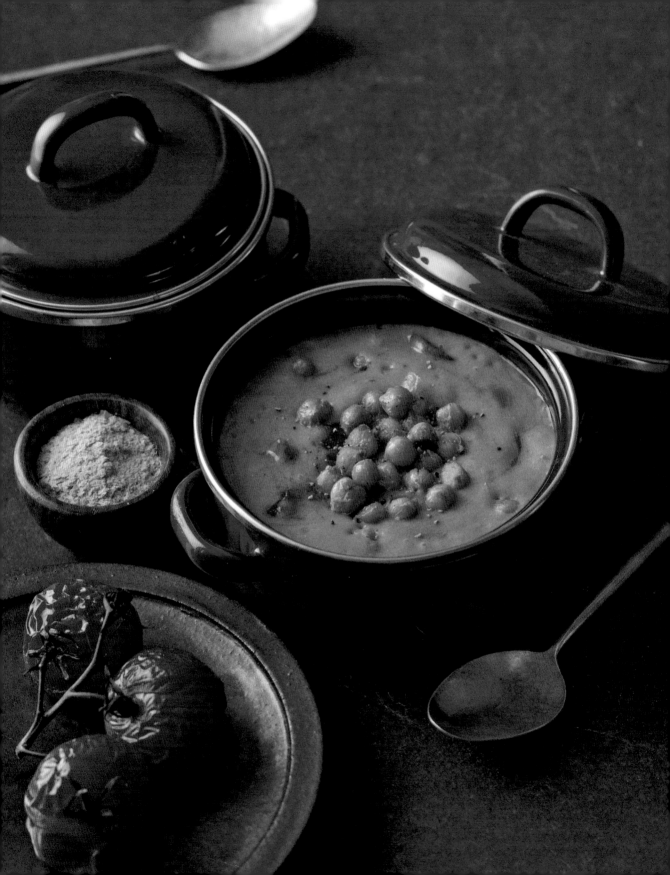

Enrich Me:
ITALIAN ROASTED TOMATO AND CHICKPEA

MAKES 6 SERVINGS (SERVING SIZE: 1½ CUPS)

V Vegan   **GF** Gluten-free

Rich and nourishing chickpeas provide fiber, protein, and a host of vitamins to keep your body in tip-top shape. Plus, this soup contains nutritional yeast, which delivers a cheesy flavor with a healthful dose of energizing vitamin B$_{12}$.

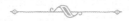

Preheat the oven to 425°F.

Place the tomatoes on a baking sheet lined with parchment paper. Drizzle with 1 tablespoon of oil and lightly season with salt and pepper. Roast for 30 minutes, or until softened.

In a large pot, warm the remaining 1 tablespoon oil over medium heat. Add the onion and garlic and sauté for 3 to 5 minutes. Mix in the tomatoes, chickpeas, broth, basil, cumin, paprika, and nutritional yeast and bring to a boil. Reduce heat to low and simmer until chickpeas are tender, about 30 minutes, then remove from heat. Reserve 2 cups of the soup, set aside, and transfer the rest to a high-powered blender. Puree until smooth and then combine the mixtures, season with salt and pepper, and serve.

8 Roma tomatoes, halved

2 tablespoons extra-virgin olive oil

Himalayan or sea salt and freshly ground black pepper

1 medium yellow onion, chopped

3 cloves garlic, minced

4½ cups cooked chickpeas, no salt added

4 cups low-sodium vegetable broth

2 tablespoons minced fresh basil

1 teaspoon ground cumin

½ teaspoon paprika

6 tablespoons nutritional yeast

Power Up!

ADD TO YOUR POT ALONG WITH THE OTHER SPICES:

½ teaspoon ground turmeric (stir in with other spices)

½ teaspoon ground cayenne pepper (stir in with other spices)

MEAL MATH per serving						
calories	*fat*	*sodium*	*carbs*	*fiber*	*sugar*	*protein*
300	6g	160mg	44g	11g	5g	14g

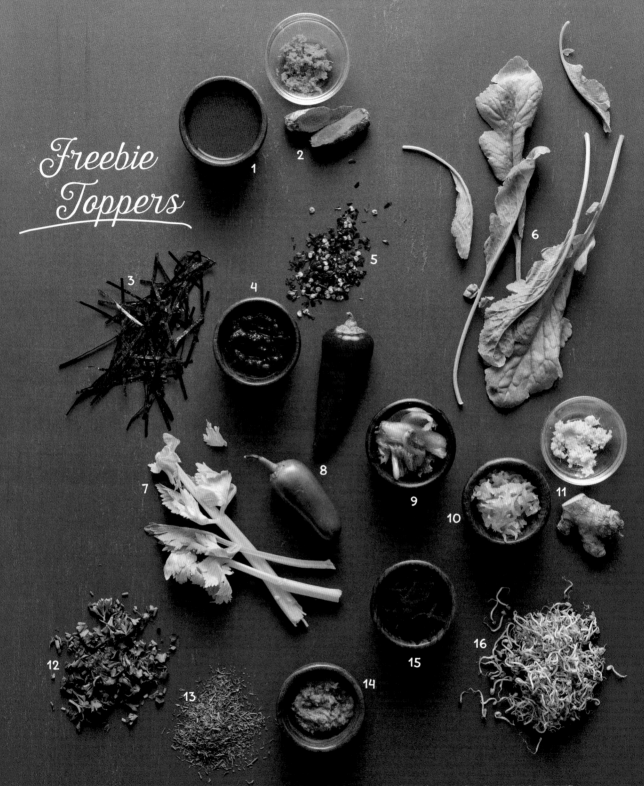

Freebie Toppers

FREEBIE TOPPERS: 1. HOT SAUCE; 2. TURMERIC ROOT; 3. DRIED NORI FLAKES; 4. HARISSA PASTE;
5. RED PEPPER FLAKES; 6. WATERCRESS; 7. CELERY LEAVES; 8. CHILI PEPPERS; 9. KIMCHI;
10. SAUERKRAUT; 11. GINGER ROOT; 12. FRESH HERBS (PARSLEY, CILANTRO); 13. DRIED HERBS;
14. HORSERADISH; 15. SHREDDED BEETS; 16. BROCCOLI SPROUTS

Power Up: Savory Soup Toppers

Craving an extra hit of heat or a little bit of crunch in your savory soups? Feel free to add some pep to your souping step with any of these toppers. I didn't throw them together willy-nilly—just like the breakfast toppings, studies suggest serious health-boosting properties in all the ingredients below. So read (and add) on!

1. Freebie Toppers: Be Liberal!

NOT JUST FLAVOR: WHY THESE FOODS POWER UP YOUR MEAL

Basil: All hail the king! Basil is considered "the king of herbs" for good reason. This fragrant leaf enhances the taste of almost anything, plus it contains antioxidant flavonoids as well as antimicrobial and anti-inflammatory oils.

Shredded beets: You know what the deep red ruby color of beets means? They're a jewel of a root, chock-full of betalains—compounds with potent anti-inflammatory actions. Keep to a tablespoon or less.

Black pepper: Put some pep in your soup! Not only does it add a flavor kick, but black pepper also contains piperine, which has antioxidant properties and possible antitumor effects. Plus, when used in conjunction with turmeric, it enhances curcumin absorbtion (the nutrient found in turmeric) by up to 2,000 percent!

Broccoli sprouts: Step aside and make way for our VIP A-list star. Just 1 tablespoon of broccoli sprouts contains as much sulforaphane (a cancer-fighting phytochemical) as 1 pound of mature broccoli!

Cayenne pepper: Burn, fat, burn! Cayenne's spiciness comes from capsaicin, a powerful compound that research shows may not only help burn fat but also combat cardiovascular disease and cancer.

Celery leaves: Don't toss them out—they contain at least five times as much calcium as the stalk! These luscious leaves add so much more than flavor and chew to your meal.

Chives: Onions too intense for your dishes? Keep calm and chive on! Chives have a more mellow taste than onions yet still contain a wealth of nutrients, including phytochemicals with potential cancer-fighting properties.

Cilantro: This sweet and tasty herb is a great source of iron and magnesium, which may help fight anemia. Studies have shown it may have antibiotic, anti-inflammatory, and detoxifying properties.

Coriander seeds: Dried coriander fruits, or coriander seeds, have a wonderful nutty citrus flavor. I love them for their potential to lower cholesterol and their supreme antioxidant capabilities.

Cumin: A spice that gives Mexican food its distinctive flavor without the salt content, cumin is packed with iron and has been shown to help with diabetes, cardiovascular disease, and asthmatic conditions.

Dill: Dill's natural qualities can help clean your insides. This herb is known to have antioxidant properties as well as calcium and iron.

Ginger: This dazzling root doesn't just impart great flavor to your soup, it's also a very powerful digestion aid and anti-inflammatory compound. It also may increase satiety (the feeling of fullness) after a meal!

Harissa paste: A spicy chile paste that's used in North African and Middle Eastern dishes, harissa typically contains chile peppers; garlic; tomatoes; olive oil; lemon juice; and spices such as cumin, coriander, caraway, and mint. Talk about some concentrated antioxidant and anti-inflammatory effects!

Horseradish: Contains more glucosinolates—code for cancer-fighting phytochemicals—than most cruciferous vegetables out there. Evidence demonstrates that these compounds may help lower your risk of cancer. Plus the intense taste of this spicy root will give your meal a huge kick.

Jalapeños: Feeling hot, hot, hot! Fun fact: The hotter the pepper, the more capsaicin it contains, which means higher potential to fight against cancer by acting as an anti-inflammatory and antioxidant agent. Bring on that burn!

Kimchi: Now that's what I call Seoul food! This traditional Korean delicacy is made by fermenting cabbage with healthful probiotics then seasoning with other anti-inflammatory and fat-burning foods. Research suggests that kimchi may have anticancer, antiobesity, probiotic, cholesterol-reducing, antiaging, brain health, and immunity-enhancing properties.

Lime: Squirt some lime for a fresh, zingy boost of vitamin C! And don't throw out the peel—just like a lemon peel, the lime peel contains limonene and other compounds that have potent antioxidant effects!

Mint: Mint does so much more than freshen up your breath! Studies show that this invigorating and cooling herb may relieve pain, support your immune system, act as an antimicrobial agent, and even calm an upset stomach.

Mustard seeds: Studies have shown these little guys may fight cancer. They're a great source of selenium, an essential mineral that works as an antioxidant to protect your body's cells.

Nori: Need a nutrition fix? Just say nori! Seaweed is a nutritional superstar with a variety of minerals that may even protect against cancer. And at only fifteen to twenty cents a sheet, it's the real deal for a steal!

Nutritional yeast: Don't let the name throw you off. This ingredient is a delicious, healthful flavor stand-in for cheese, and it supplies vitamin B_{12}, which the body uses to produce energy. And with no salt, no sugar, and no cholesterol, nutritional yeast will keep you saying yes, yes, yes!

Oregano: The spice that's synonymous with Italian flavoring boasts a huge amount of antioxidants. Oregano also contains carnosol and quercetin, which may have powerful anticancer properties. And just a little goes a long way, so all you need is a pinch!

Parsley: Meet my secret red-carpet-ready trick! Parsley is a great debloater that helps flush excess water out of the body and is loaded with vitamins and minerals. I refer to parsley as a multivitamin, so go ahead and "sprig" into action!

Red pepper flakes: Some like it hot—and you should, too. Red pepper flakes (from the same plant as cayenne pepper) get their kick from capsaicin, a powerful compound that may not only help burn fat away but also fights cardiovascular disease and cancer.

Rosemary: Along with its substantial iron and calcium content, this herb has potent anti-inflammatory and DNA-protecting properties. The antioxidants in rosemary may also have cancer-fighting capabilities, even in the small amounts used in cooking!

Sauerkraut: Literally meaning "sour cabbage," sauerkraut produces compounds that may prevent cancer growth. It's also packed with healthful probiotics, but just watch the amount you're using because it tends to be high in sodium.

Shallots: Think of shallots as the sweeter cousin of onions. Shallots are great for their potential anti-inflammatory and anticancer effects and help bring both flavor and flavonoids to your plate!

Turmeric: An ever-growing body of research continues to show that curcumin, the main compound in turmeric, has impressive antioxidant and anti-inflammatory effects that may help fight against a wide range of cancers as well as cardiovascular disease. Just a pinch can have a huge effect in protecting your cells from damage!

Watercress: Mirror, mirror, on the wall, who's the most nutrient-dense veggie to rule them all? It's watercress! Just 1 cup and 4 calories (fewer than half a stick of gum) will give you 106 percent of your daily vitamin K, 24 percent of your vitamin C, and 22 percent of your vitamin A needs. Plus it's rich in indole-3-carbinol, which may fight cancer.

2. Fat Toppers

Although they are natural and satisfying, use with discretion!

Topper	Calories per Tablespoon (tsp)	Topper	Calories per Tablespoon (tsp)
Oils (chili, olive, walnut, avocado oil)	120 (40)	Nuts (almonds, walnuts, pecans)	30–50 (12–17)
Tahini	90 (30)	Pepitas	40 (13)
Avocado	¼ fruit = 60	Sesame seeds	45 (15)
Pine nuts	60 (20)	Powerfood Pesto (page 204)	40 (13)
Hemp	53 (18)	Sesame Kale Pesto (page 203)	25 (8)
Sunflower seeds	46 (15)	Cashew Crème (page 206)	60 (60)

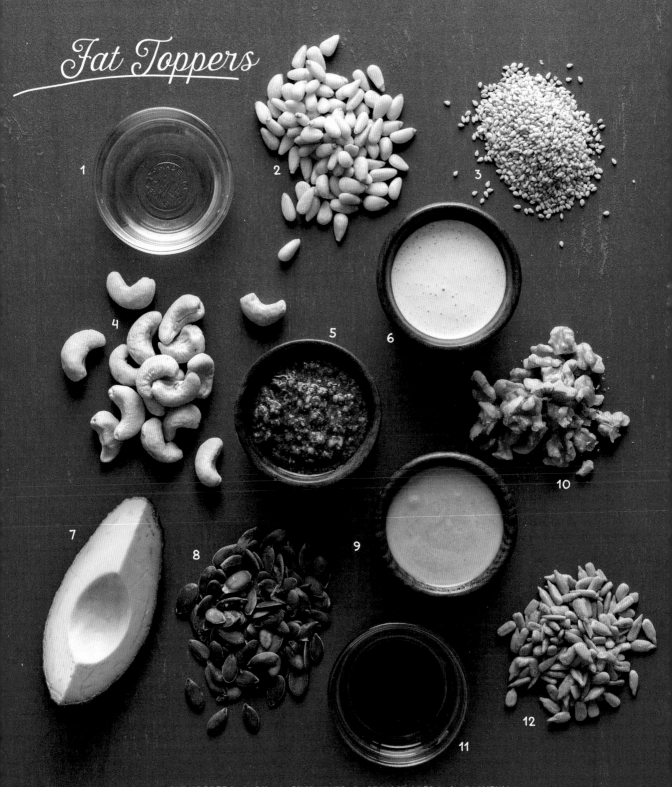

Fat Toppers

FAT TOPPERS: 1. OIL; 2. PINE NUTS; 3. SESAME SEEDS; 4. CASHEWS;
5. PESTO; 6. TAHINI; 7. AVOCADO; 8. PEPITAS; 9. CASHEW CRÈME; 10. WALNUTS;
11. CHILI OIL; 12. SUNFLOWER SEEDS

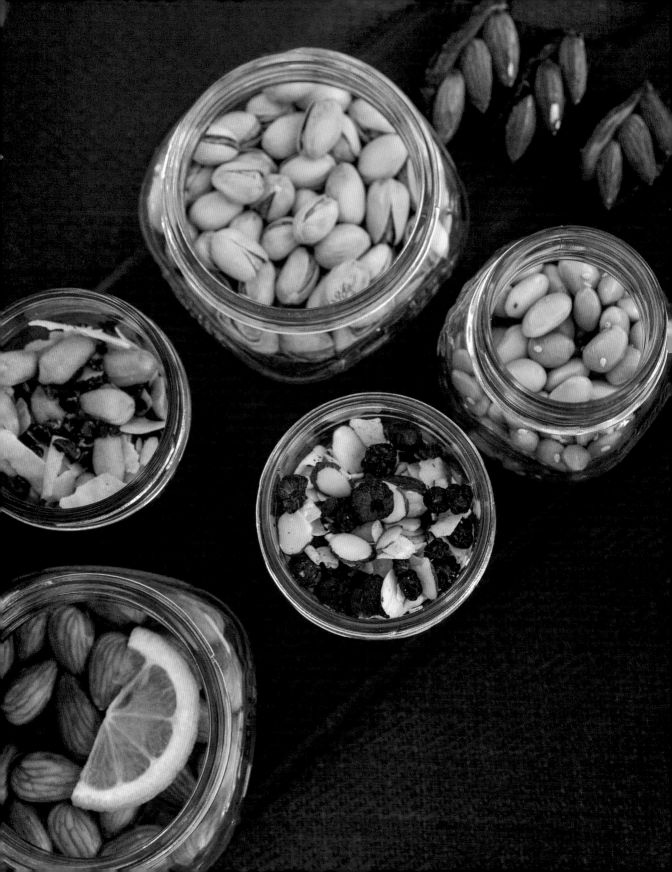

Snack Time

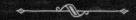

Your P.M. snack is mandatory—but I'm making it as simple as possible, with no-cook, blend-and-go recipes that come together in a flash. You'll also find soups that you can cook up in a batch. Make a big pot or two on Sunday so you'll have nourishing, ready-to-go snacks set for the rest of the week.

Chill-and-Go Snack Soups

I get it; that little thing we call life gets hectic and you don't always have the time to simmer a pot of soup on the stove. My chill-and-go snack soups are wholesome, and, while simple in strategy, are every bit as nutritious and tasty as their cooked counterparts. Quick, easy, and refreshing; these clean-eating snacks fit the bill calorically and will hold you over until your next meal.

Invigorate Me:
SPANISH RED PEPPER

MAKES 4 SERVINGS (SERVING SIZE: 1 CUP)

V *Vegan* **GF** *Gluten-free*

Place the tomatoes, bell peppers, garlic, vinegar, oil, and lemon juice in a high-powered blender and puree until smooth. Season with salt and pepper to taste. Chill before serving.

4 large tomatoes, chopped

3 medium red bell peppers, cored, seeded, and chopped

1 to 2 cloves garlic, chopped

4 tablespoons red wine vinegar

2 tablespoons extra-virgin olive oil

3 tablespoons freshly squeezed lemon juice

Himalayan or sea salt and freshly ground black pepper

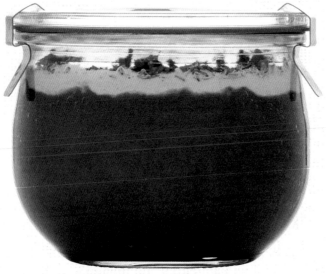

Power Up!

TOP WITH OR BLEND IN:

1 teaspoon Cashew Crème (page 206)

1 tablespoon chopped fresh cilantro or parsley

2 diced cucumbers

MEAL MATH per serving						
calories	fat	sodium	carbs	fiber	sugar	protein
140	8g	15mg	16g	5g	10g	3g

Endless Summer:
CUCUMBER AVOCADO

MAKES 4 SERVINGS (SERVING SIZE: 1 CUP)

VO *Vegan option* **GF** *Gluten-free*

1 ripe avocado

2 medium cucumbers, chopped

1 cup organic plain 2% Greek yogurt or Vegan Yogurt (page 135)

3 tablespoons chopped fresh chives

Juice of ½ lime

½ serrano pepper, seeded and chopped, or pinch of ground cayenne pepper

8 ice cubes

Himalayan or sea salt and freshly ground black pepper

Chopped cherry tomatoes, for garnish (optional)

Power Up!

TOP WITH OR BLEND IN:

1 teaspoon nutritional yeast

Place the avocado, cucumbers, yogurt, chives, lime juice, serrano pepper, and ice cubes in a high-powered blender and puree until smooth. Season with salt and pepper to taste. Chill before serving, and if using, garnish with tomatoes.

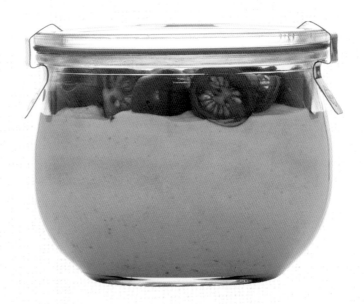

MEAL MATH per serving						
calories	fat	sodium	carbs	fiber	sugar	protein
140	9g	25mg	9g	4g	4g	7g

Purple Potion:
SUCCULENT BERRY

MAKES 1 SERVING

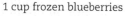 Vegan **GF** *Gluten-free*

Place the blueberries, milk, date, and ice cubes in a high-powered blender and blend away. Top with the coconut flakes, if using.

1 cup frozen blueberries

1 cup unsweetened plant-based milk (see page 139)

1 date, pitted

3 ice cubes

1 tablespoon unsweetened coconut flakes, for garnish (optional)

Power Up!

TOP WITH OR BLEND IN:

1 teaspoon blackberry, pomegranate, acai, or raspberry Powerfood Powder (see page 58)

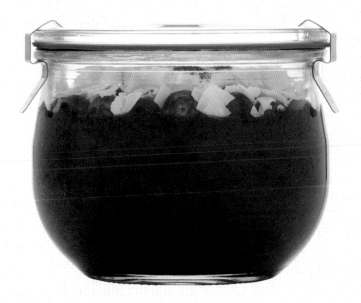

MEAL MATH per serving						
calories	fat	sodium	carbs	fiber	sugar	protein
140	5g	150mg	25g	7g	16g	0g

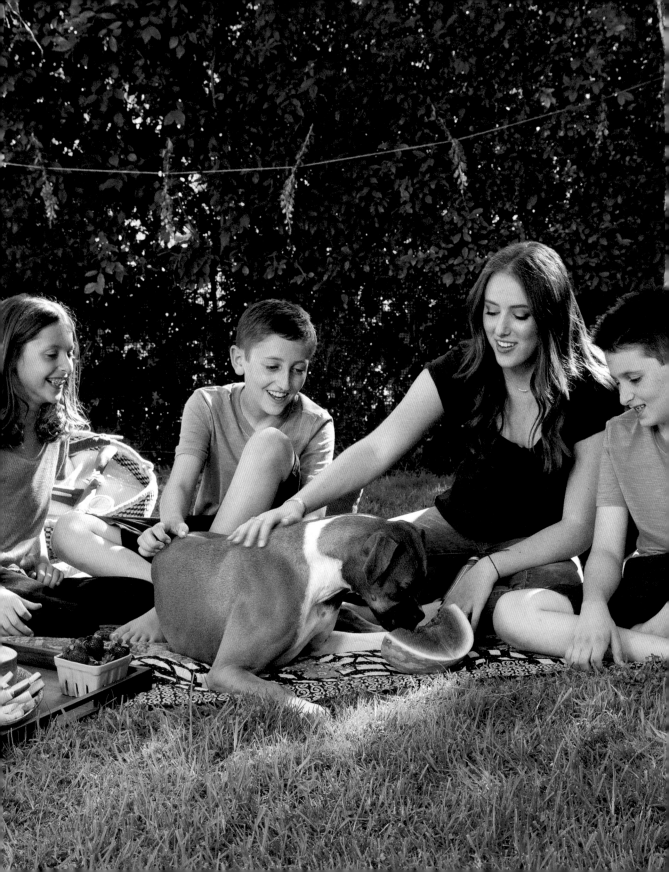

Soothe Me:
BLUEBERRY SPICE

MAKES 1 SERVING

V Vegan   **GF** Gluten-free

Combine the milk, chia seeds, blueberries, cinnamon, and maple syrup, if using, in a mason jar. Shake, let sit overnight in the refrigerator, and you're ready to go!

1 cup unsweetened plant-based milk (see page 139)

1 tablespoon chia seeds

½ cup fresh or frozen blueberries

¼ teaspoon cinnamon

½ teaspoon pure maple syrup (optional)

Power Up!

TOP WITH OR STIR IN:

1 teaspoon blueberry Powerfood Powder (see page 58)

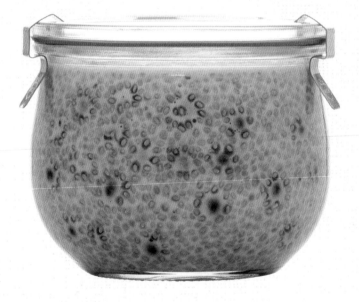

MEAL MATH *per serving*						
calories	*fat*	*sodium*	*carbs*	*fiber*	*sugar*	*protein*
170	10g	200mg	13g	8g	7g	4g

Blush: RASPBERRY KEFIR

MAKES 1 SERVING

GF *Gluten-free*

½ cup organic plain 2% kefir

½ cup unsweetened
plant-based milk (see page 139)

2 teaspoons chia seeds

½ cup frozen raspberries

1 teaspoon raw honey (optional)

Power Up!

TOP WITH OR STIR IN:

1 teaspoon raspberry Powerfood
Powder (see page 58)

Combine the kefir, milk, chia seeds, raspberries, and raw honey, if using, in a mason jar. Shake, and let sit for a few hours (or overnight) in the refrigerator, and you're ready to go!

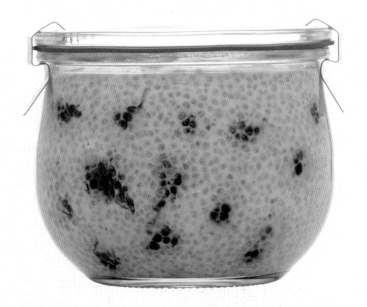

MEAL MATH per serving						
calories	fat	sodium	carbs	fiber	sugar	protein
160	7g	170mg	14g	8g	9g	8g

Lush: ACAI BANANA

MAKES 1 SERVING

V *Vegan* **GF** *Gluten-free*

Place the acai pack, ice cubes, banana, and water in a high-powered blender and blend away. Sprinkle the almonds on top, if using.

1 acai pack (found at a health food store) or 1 teaspoon acai Powerfood Powder (see page 58)

3 ice cubes

1 small frozen banana

½ cup filtered water

1 teaspoon sliced almonds, for garnish (optional)

Power Up!

TOP WITH OR BLEND IN:

¼ teaspoon granulated orange peel

½ teaspoon Ceylon cinnamon

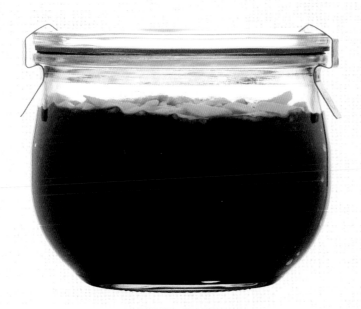

MEAL MATH per serving						
calories	*fat*	*sodium*	*carbs*	*fiber*	*sugar*	*protein*
160	5g	25mg	27g	6g	12g	1g

Chop and Simmer Snack Soups

These straight-forward soup-erb recipes will fill your bowl with an impressive depth of flavor. Make room in your fridge—one batch will make enough for several snacking occasions.

Turnip the Beets:
RUBY ROOT SOUP

MAKES 6 SERVINGS (SERVING SIZE: 1 CUP)

V *Vegan* **GF** *Gluten-free*

Beets can't be beat! Their powerful anti-inflammatory qualities give this juicy red soup a real nutritional boost—just a single beet does the trick. Once you add in a pinch of antioxidant-rich oregano and plump vitamin-loaded tomatoes, the result is a vibrant, refreshing, mildly sweet detox you can stir with a spoon. Plus, you can serve it up hot or chilled—either way, this dish is a total gem.

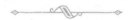

Heat the oil in a large pot over medium heat. Add the onion and garlic and sauté for 3 to 5 minutes. Add the carrots, celery, turnip, beet, tomatoes, tomato paste, broth, and oregano and bring to a boil. Reduce the heat and simmer, covered, for 15 to 20 minutes, until the veggies are tender but not mushy. If using, stir in the kale and season with salt and pepper to taste and serve.

See photo on page 16.

1 tablespoon extra-virgin olive oil

1 small onion, chopped

2 cloves garlic, minced

2 medium carrots, chopped

2 stalks celery, chopped

1 medium turnip, chopped

1 large beet, peeled and chopped

1 cup diced tomatoes

1 tablespoon tomato paste

4 cups low-sodium vegetable broth

1 teaspoon dried oregano

2 cups chopped kale (optional)

Himalayan or sea salt and freshly ground black pepper

Power Up!

ADD TO YOUR BOWL:

1 to 2 tablespoons chopped fresh parsley

1 tablespoon Cashew Crème (page 206) or 2 tablespoons organic plain 2% Greek yogurt

MEAL MATH per serving						
calories	fat	sodium	carbs	fiber	sugar	protein
60	3g	150mg	9g	3g	4g	2g

Focus Me:
CHILLED CARROT AND DILL

MAKES 6 SERVINGS (SERVING SIZE: 1 CUP)

V *Vegan*   **GF** *Gluten-free*

1 tablespoon extra-virgin olive oil

1 medium onion, chopped

½-inch piece fresh turmeric, peeled and minced, or ½ teaspoon ground

1 clove garlic, minced

Freshly ground black pepper

12 medium carrots, chopped

4 cups low-sodium vegetable broth

Himalayan or sea salt

2 tablespoons chopped fresh dill

Power Up!

ADD PROTEIN TO YOUR BOWL:

1 tablespoon hemp seeds

Whether you're craving a savory snack or something a little on the sweeter side, this soup's got you covered thanks to the carrots and abundance of fresh herbs and spices. Did you know that cooking the carrots amps up your ability to absorb the antioxidants they have to offer? But don't let this veg steal the show—dill contains 10 percent of your daily calcium quota in just 1 tablespoon, along with plenty of iron. Now that's something to hone in on.

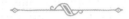

Heat the oil in a large pot over medium heat. Add the onion and sauté for 3 to 5 minutes, until softened. Stir in the turmeric and garlic and season with pepper. Add the carrots and broth and bring to a boil. Reduce the heat and simmer, covered, 20 to 30 minutes, until the carrots are tender. Add salt to taste. Remove from heat and allow the soup to cool for about 10 minutes. Carefully pour the soup into a high-powered blender and puree until smooth. Chill the soup completely. Stir in dill before serving.

See photo on page 16.

MEAL MATH per serving						
calories	fat	sodium	carbs	fiber	sugar	protein
100	3g	190mg	19g	5g	8g	2g

Restore Me:
DETOX VEGGIE

MAKES 6 SERVINGS (SERVING SIZE: 1 CUP)

V Vegan   **GF** Gluten-free

This soup has "DETOX" written all over it in big green letters! And with its abundance of fresh veggies, how could it be mistaken for anything but? It's my all-time favorite afternoon pick-me-up; it comes together in a flash so you have more time to enjoy a bowl that's bursting with wholesome, pure flavors and plenty of beneficial nutrients. If you're in the mood for a chunkier meal, skip the blending and enjoy this soup as is.

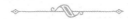

Heat the oil in a large pot over medium heat. Add the onion, garlic, and ginger and sauté for 3 to 5 minutes, until softened. Add the broccoli, spinach, parsnips, celery, and parsley and continue cooking until the spinach wilts, about 1 to 2 minutes. Pour in just enough broth to cover the vegetables (you may not use all of it) and simmer, covered, until the vegetables are soft, about 20 minutes. Carefully pour the soup into a high-powered blender and puree until smooth. Return the soup to the pot and season with salt and pepper to taste.

See photo on page 16.

1 tablespoon extra-virgin olive oil

1 medium onion, chopped

2 cloves garlic, minced

1-inch piece fresh ginger, peeled and chopped

4 cups broccoli florets

3 cups baby spinach

2 parsnips, chopped

2 stalks celery, chopped

3 tablespoons chopped fresh parsley

½ cup low-sodium vegetable broth

Himalayan or sea salt and freshly ground black pepper

Power Up!

ADD TO YOUR BOWL:

1 tablespoon pine nuts

1 tablespoon chopped fresh parsley

MEAL MATH per serving						
calories	fat	sodium	carbs	fiber	sugar	protein
100	3g	115mg	17g	6g	4g	4g

Refresh Me:
CREAMY GREEN PEA WITH MINT

MAKES 4 SERVINGS (SERVING SIZE: 1 CUP)

V *Vegan* **GF** *Gluten-free*

1 tablespoon extra-virgin olive oil

½ cup chopped leeks (white parts only)

1 large shallot, chopped

3 cloves garlic, minced

3 cups low-sodium vegetable broth

3 cups frozen green peas

¼ cup chopped fresh mint

Himalayan or sea salt and freshly ground black pepper

Power Up!

ADD TO YOUR BOWL:

Fresh mint leaves

If you find yourself caught in the middle of a snack attack, try something that's both sweet and savory to satisfy your craving. This refreshing snack is not your ordinary pea soup—it has a refreshing and invigorating flavor due to the mint. Fresh mint is not only a breath freshener—studies show that this cooling herb may relieve pain, support your immune system, and even calm an upset stomach. So get the hint and add some mint!

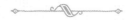

Heat the oil in a large pot over medium heat. Add the leeks, shallot, and garlic and sauté about 3 or 5 minutes, until tender. Add the broth and bring to a boil. Stir in the peas, reduce the heat, and simmer, covered, until the peas are warmed through, 5 to 7 minutes. Remove from heat, add the mint, and season with salt and pepper to taste. Carefully pour the soup into a high-powered blender and puree until smooth, then pour back into the pot and serve.

See photo on page 16.

MEAL MATH per serving						
calories	fat	sodium	carbs	fiber	sugar	protein
150	4g	115mg	22g	7g	8g	7g

Goddess:
VEGAN CREAM OF MUSHROOM

MAKES 3 SERVINGS (SERVING SIZE: 1 CUP)

V Vegan **GF** Gluten-free

Feast your eyes . . . and stomach! This is my take on a big bowl of creamy mushroom soup. It's every bit as comforting and satisfying as the kind you're used to but is a cinch to whip up and checks out much higher in the nutrition department. I'm a big fan of mushrooms—they're high in protein and have tons of biologically active compounds that have may keep cancer, diabetes, and cholesterol at bay.

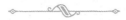

Heat the oil in a large pot over medium heat. Add the leeks and garlic and sauté for 2 to 3 minutes. Stir in the mushrooms and cook for another 2 minutes. If desired, reserve ½ cup of the sautéed mushrooms and set aside for a Power Up topping (at right). Add the wine, if using. Add the plant-based milk and bring to a boil. Reduce the heat and simmer, covered, for 20 minutes. Carefully pour the soup into a high-powered blender and pulse three or four times, until mixed but not completely smooth. Season with salt and pepper to taste and serve.

See photo on page 16.

1 tablespoon extra-virgin olive oil

½ cup chopped leeks

1 clove garlic, minced

4½ cups mushrooms, sliced (any variety)

Splash of dry white wine (optional)

1½ cups unsweetened plant-based milk (see page 139)

Himalayan or sea salt and freshly ground black pepper

Power Up!

ADD TO YOUR BOWL:

½ cup chopped watercress

½ cup sautéed mushrooms (reserved from recipe)

MEAL MATH per serving						
calories	fat	sodium	carbs	fiber	sugar	protein
100	6g	95mg	10g	3g	1g	3g

Robust Tomato:
ROASTED TOMATO BASIL

MAKES 4 SERVINGS (SERVING SIZE: 1 CUP)

V Vegan **GF** Gluten-free

8 Roma tomatoes, quartered

1 medium onion, sliced

2 tablespoons extra-virgin olive oil

2 tablespoons minced fresh basil

Himalayan or sea salt and freshly ground black pepper

4 cloves garlic

3 cups low-sodium vegetable broth

3 tablespoons tomato paste

1 teaspoon pure maple syrup, to reduce acidity (optional)

Power Up!

ADD TO YOUR BOWL:

Fresh basil leaves

The color red symbolizes power, and this savory soup is no exception. Roasting the tomatoes gives them an incredible depth of flavor—and actually allows your body to absorb even more of the almighty anti-oxidant lycopene than when they're raw. With a pinch of fragrant basil, an impressive antimicrobial and antioxidant, this soup will give you the nutritional punch you need to power through your day.

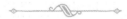

Preheat the oven to 375°F.

Spread the tomatoes and onion onto a parchment-lined baking sheet. Toss with the oil and basil and sprinkle with salt and pepper. Tuck the garlic cloves into the tomato wedges so they won't burn. Roast for 40 minutes, until the tomatoes have shrunk to half their size and are lightly browned.

Meanwhile, warm the broth in a large pot over medium heat. Stir in the tomato paste. Add the roasted veggies and bring the soup to a boil. Reduce the heat and simmer, covered, for 8 to 10 minutes. Pour the soup into a high-powered blender and puree until smooth. Stir in the maple syrup, if using. Season with salt and pepper to taste and serve.

MEAL MATH per serving						
calories	fat	sodium	carbs	fiber	sugar	protein
140	8g	15mg	16g	5g	3g	10g

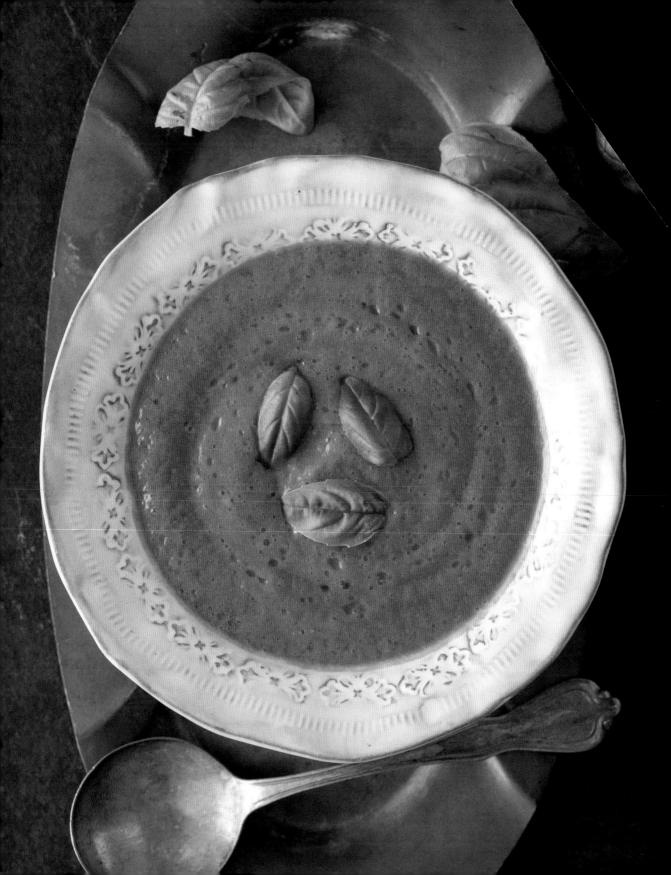

Freebie Soups

Yes, you read that right: freebie! I want you to use these soups to carry you over in case you want something extra.

Turn any of these freebies into a complete meal by topping with a protein, healthful fat (see pages 162–163), and of course, a Power Up for an extra nutritional punch.

STEP 1: SAUTÉ THE AROMATICS.

Heat 1 tablespoon high-quality oil in a large pot over medium heat. Add 1 cup chopped onion, leeks, or shallots. Then add 1 to 2 cloves minced garlic and sauté 3 to 5 minutes, until softened.

STEP 2: CHOOSE YOUR FREEBIE FLAVOR.

Add the ingredients—including the broth of your choice—to the aromatic base. The end result is up to you: Feel free to blend away or leave your soup chunky. These veg-packed and super-low-cal bowls will support your daily dose of detox without compromising your waistline goals. And they come together in just two simple steps.

Immunity: MUSHROOM ARTICHOKE

Turn the heat to low and add 2 chopped carrots, 4 cups sliced mushrooms, ⅛ teaspoon each dried rosemary and thyme (or ½ teaspoon fresh rosemary and thyme, minced) and cook, covered, 10 to 12 minutes, until carrots are tender, stirring frequently. Add 4 cups broth and 2 cups frozen artichoke hearts and bring the soup to a boil. Turn off the heat and stir in 1 tablespoon freshly squeezed lemon juice, 3 cups baby spinach, and 1 tablespoon nutritional yeast (optional). Season with salt and pepper to taste and serve.

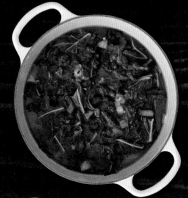

Clean: SPINACH AND KALE

Add 2 cups chopped kale, 4 cups broth, and a pinch of red pepper flakes and bring the soup to a boil. Lower heat and simmer, covered, until the kale is tender, 6 to 8 minutes. Add 3 cups baby spinach (for an ultra-detox, add a handful of watercress) and simmer 2 more minutes. Season with salt and pepper to taste and serve.

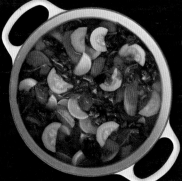

Revive Me: HOLY MINESTRONE

Add 2 chopped yellow squash, 2 chopped zucchini, and 1 chopped carrot and sauté for 5 minutes, until softened. Add 3 chopped tomatoes and 8 cups broth and bring to a boil. Reduce the heat and simmer, covered, 10 to 15 minutes. Stir in 2 cups chopped kale and simmer about 5 minutes. Add 2 cups baby spinach and simmer another 2 minutes. Season with salt and pepper to taste and serve.

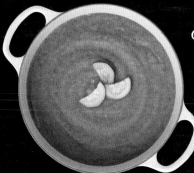

Purify: ZUCCHINI

Add 6 medium sliced zucchini, reduce the heat to low, and sauté 5 to 7 minutes, until softened. Add enough broth to cover the zucchini (about 3 cups), cover, and simmer 20 minutes. Ladle the vegetable mixture and 1 cup broth into a high-powered blender and puree until smooth, gradually adding remaining broth to reach desired consistency. Season with salt and pepper to taste and serve.

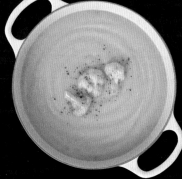

Curried Away: CURRY CAULIFLOWER

Add 6 cups cauliflower florets and 3 cups broth and simmer, covered, 15 to 20 minutes. Remove lid, reduce the heat to medium-low, and cook 15 to 20 minutes more. Stir in 2 teaspoons curry powder and ½ teaspoon ground turmeric. Carefully pour the soup into a high-powered blender and puree until smooth. Season with salt and pepper to taste and serve.

No-Brainer Soups

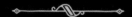

When you're having a crazy week and are pressed for time, these soups eliminate all the guesswork and equip you with the essentials to make a delicious made-from-scratch meal. These recipes are a blank canvas—simply toss any low-starch veg you have on hand into a pot of broth for a Freebie Soup. Or you can add a protein and fat of your choice to make it a complete meal! Also, using leftover Simple Roasted Veg (see page 193) will introduce a whole new level of complex flavor to your taste buds.

EFFORTLESS BASE SOUP

For the soup: Pour any amount of broth into a pot. Heat it up and toss in whatever low-starch veg that you have on hand—fresh, frozen, or prechopped—to make this super quick. Bring the pot to a boil and then simmer for 10 minutes or until vegetables are tender. My favorite veg to include for max detox are anti-inflammatory mushrooms and cancer-crushing cruciferous broccoli, cabbage, cauliflower, or bok choy.

Make it a meal: Add protein of your choice and top with a fat, and your meal is a done deal!

OPTIONAL TWISTS
FOR A WHOLE NEW FLAVOR PROFILE, TRY THESE VARIATIONS:

Basic Red

Add to the broth: 1 tablespoon tomato paste (from a BPA-free container) and 4 medium tomatoes, chopped.

    Then add in your low-starch veg and cook according to the same instructions as for Effortless Base Soup. I like to add 2 cups each shredded savoy cabbage, chopped green beans, and chopped carrots—plus a handful of chopped fresh herbs, like basil.

Basic Ginger

Add to the broth: 4 tablespoons fresh ginger, peeled and chopped.

    Then add in your low-starch veg and cook according to the same instructions as for Effortless Base Soup. My suggestion: 2 cups each sliced mushrooms, shredded Chinese cabbage, and baby bok choy.

RACHEL'S ROASTED VEG SOUP

MAKES 3 SERVINGS (SERVING SIZE: 1 CUP)

V Vegan   **GF** Gluten-free

Take 3 cups Simple Roasted Veg (page 193) and toss in a high-powered blender with 1 to 1½ cups broth. In general, a good rule of thumb is a 2:1 ratio of veg to broth. Blend until smooth.

Make it a meal: Add protein of your choice and top with a fat and your meal is a done deal!

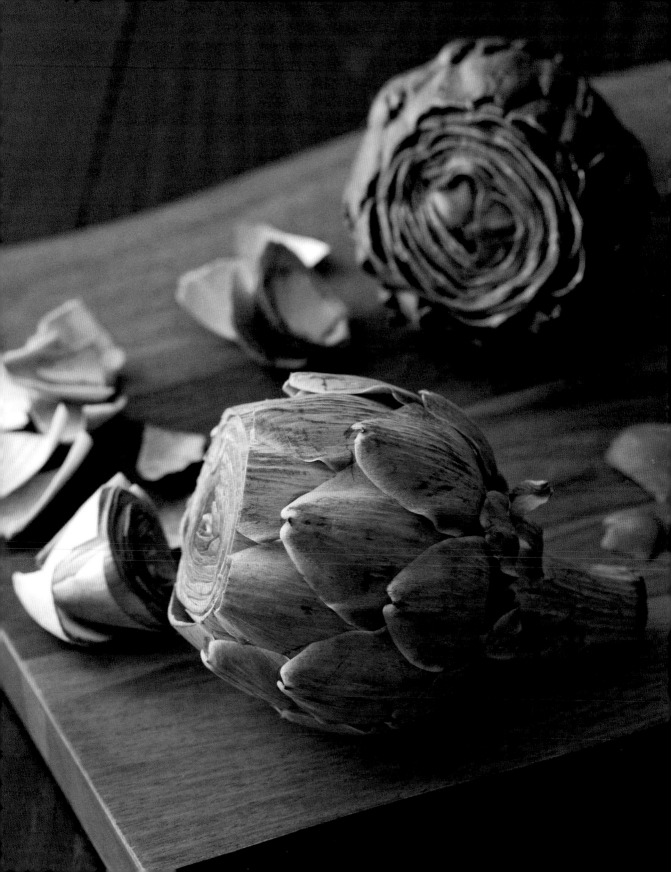

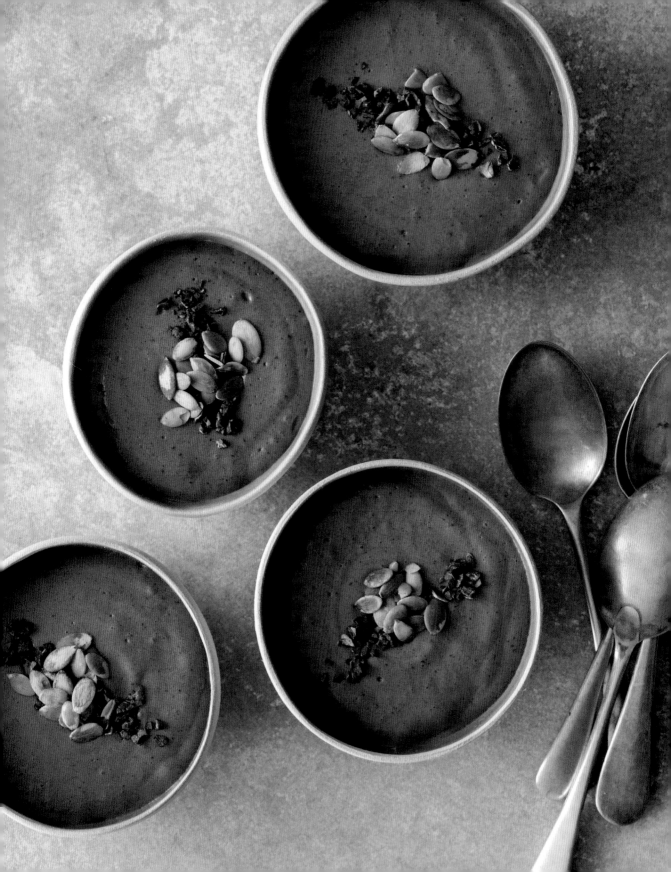

Dessert

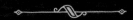

Treats? On a fast-track detox plan? Yes, you read that right! Each of these sweets fits my nutrition guidelines—which means that if you're really craving something extra after dinner (and if you're on my 24-Day Transformation), you can choose to indulge with a sweet treat knowing that it's wholesome yet still decadent enough to hit the spot.

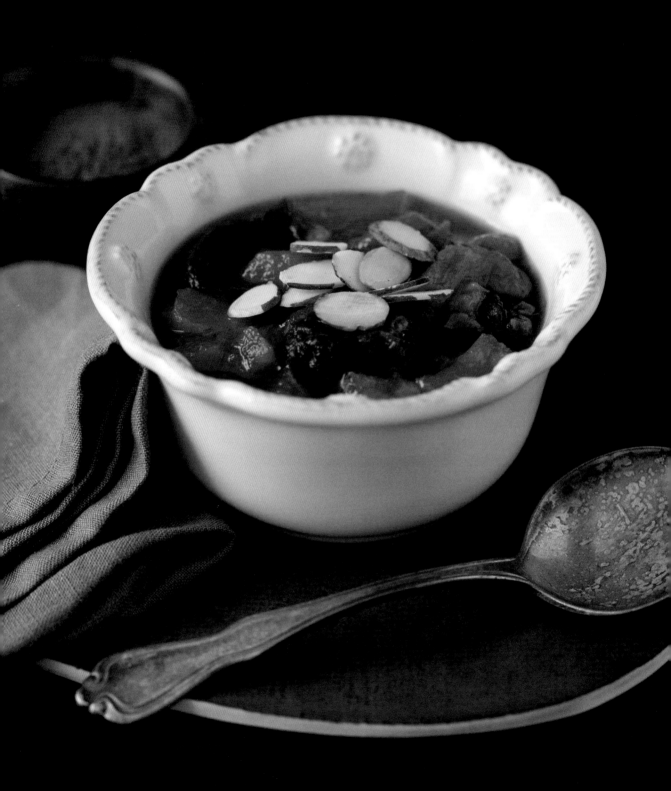

Gratify Me:
APRICOT PLUM REFRESHER

MAKES 6 TO 8 SERVINGS (SERVING SIZE: ½ CUP)

V Vegan   **GF** Gluten-free

I love how versatile this dish is; it's delicious as either a dessert or as a snack. Top it off with some sliced almonds or just add a table-spoon of this decadent soup to your morning oatmeal with a dash of cinnamon. And if you don't consider dried plums to be the most exciting food around, consider this: They have two times the amount of antioxidants as blueberries and six times as much as fresh plums!

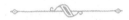

Place the apples and dried plums and apricots in a large pot and pour in the water. Bring the mixture to a boil, then reduce the heat and simmer, covered, for 1½ hours, stirring occasionally, until most of the water cooks off and the mixture thickens. Uncover and simmer for 10 to 15 minutes more. Remove from the heat and allow to cool to room temperature. Stir in the lemon juice and, if using, the chia seeds and maple syrup. Chill for at least 2 hours. Dress with the topping, if desired, before serving.

3 large green or golden apples, peeled, cored, and chopped

½ cup chopped dried sulfur-free plums

½ cup chopped dried sulfur-free apricots

3 cups filtered water

2 teaspoons freshly squeezed lemon juice

1 tablespoon chia seeds (optional)

1 tablespoon pure maple syrup (optional)

OPTIONAL TOPPING

1 tablespoon sliced almonds

MEAL MATH per serving						
calories	fat	sodium	carbs	fiber	sugar	protein
90	0g	0mg	24g	3g	18g	1g

Clarity: BERRY RICH

MAKES 4 SERVINGS (SERVING SIZE: ½ CUP)

VO *Vegan option*   **GF** *Gluten-free*

½ cup filtered water

3 cups fresh or frozen blueberries

3 cups fresh or frozen strawberries

¾ cup organic plain 2% Greek yogurt or Vegan Yogurt (page 135)

1 teaspoon grated lemon zest

3 tablespoons freshly squeezed lemon juice

1½ teaspoons ground cinnamon

1 teaspoon raw honey

OPTIONAL TOPPINGS

½ cup fresh berries of your choice

1 teaspoon cacao nibs

You don't have to surrender your sweet tooth when it comes in the form of an antioxidant fiesta. That's because this yummy berry soup features blueberries, strawberries, and lemon zest, all of which contain flavonoids to help keep your brain sharp. Even better, the superstars of this soup supply an abundance of vitamin C, so do the math and get your fill of brain food for dessert!

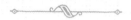

Place the water and berries in a medium saucepan over medium heat and simmer until soft, about 10 minutes. Pour the mixture into a strainer (you can reserve the antioxidant-rich liquid to flavor sparkling water for a refreshing drink), and place the berries in a high-powered blender. Add the yogurt, lemon zest, lemon juice, cinnamon, and honey. Puree until smooth, chill for at least 15 minutes, and serve. Dress with toppings, if desired.

MEAL MATH per serving						
calories	*fat*	*sodium*	*carbs*	*fiber*	*sugar*	*protein*
90	1g	15mg	19g	4g	12g	4g

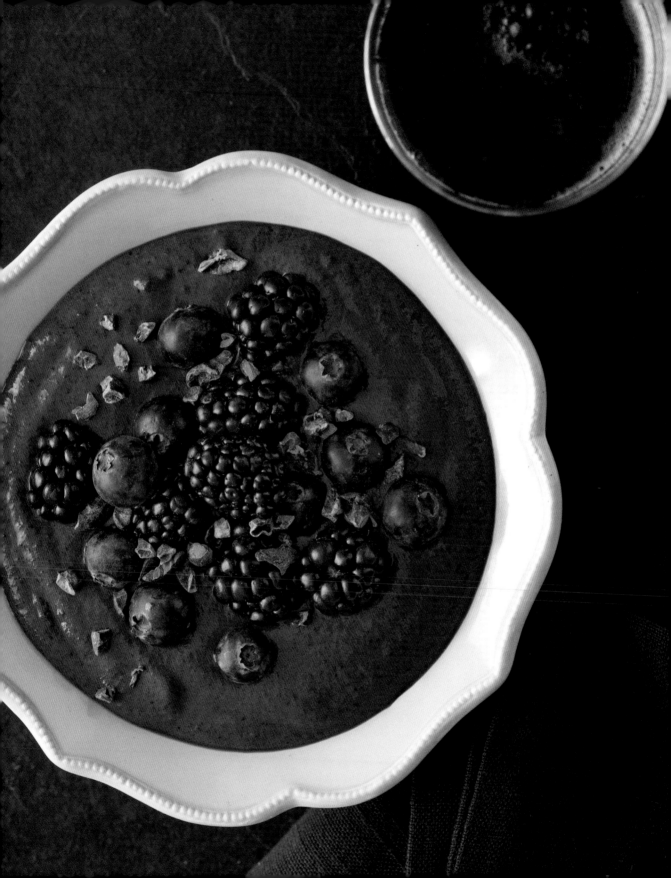

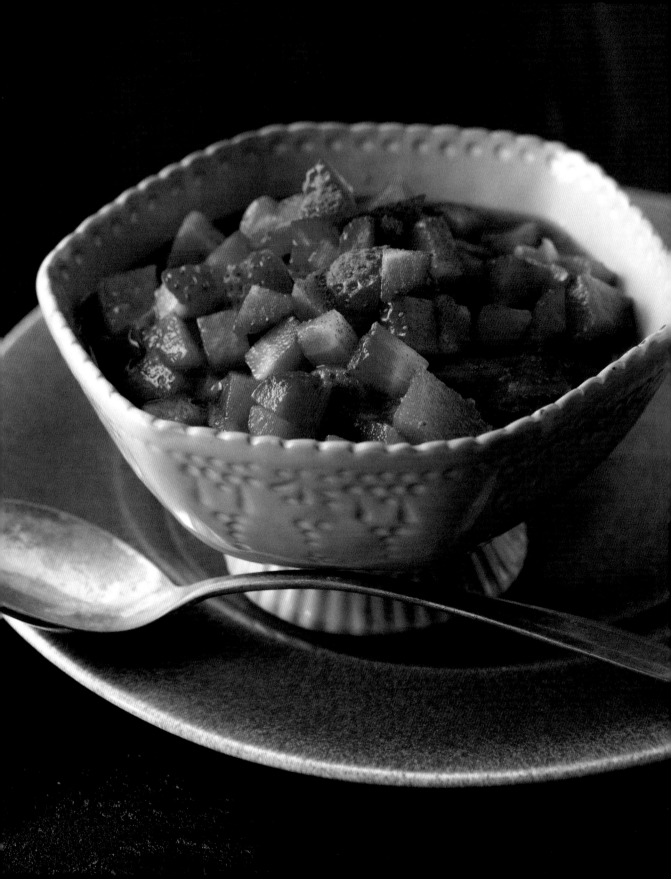

Brighten Me: PEARBERRY

MAKES 8 SERVINGS (SERVING SIZE: 1 CUP)

V Vegan   **GF** Gluten-free

Apples, pears, and strawberries—oh my! Seemingly ordinary fruits that have some extraordinary health benefits, the members in this trio deliver megadoses of vitamin C, fiber, and strong cancer-fighting antioxidants. Simmer and sip this bright bowl for dessert and then you can enjoy the leftovers as a tasty chilled breakfast soup topping or stir in ½ cup yogurt of your choice and a dash of cinnamon for a refreshing midday pick-me-up.

3 cups filtered water

3 large green apples, peeled, cored, and chopped

2 large pears, cored and chopped

3 cups fresh or frozen sliced strawberries

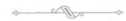

Place the water, apples, and pears in a medium pot and bring to a boil, then reduce the heat and simmer for about 45 minutes. Turn off the heat and stir in the strawberries and simmer for an additional 5 minutes. Serve either warm or chilled.

MEAL MATH per serving						
calories	fat	sodium	carbs	fiber	sugar	protein
90	0g	5mg	24g	5g	17g	<1g

Crave Me:
A DATE WITH CHOCOLATE

MAKES 1 SERVING

V *Vegan*   **GF** *Gluten-free*

½ small frozen banana

1 tablespoon raw cacao powder

½ cup unsweetened plant-based milk (see page 139)

1 date, pitted

OPTIONAL TOPPING

¼ cup fresh raspberries

You've got a hot date tonight. And trust me, it's going to be really, really good. This voluptuous combination of cacao and banana is sure to satisfy your cravings in the healthiest way possible! Dates offer a touch of natural sugar and are rich in B vitamins, minerals, and fiber, so go ahead and give yourself permission to feel decadent.

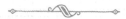

Place the banana, cacao powder, milk, and date in a high-powered blender and puree until smooth. Dress with the topping, if desired.

MEAL MATH per serving						
calories	fat	sodium	carbs	fiber	sugar	protein
110	2g	90mg	23g	5g	11g	3g

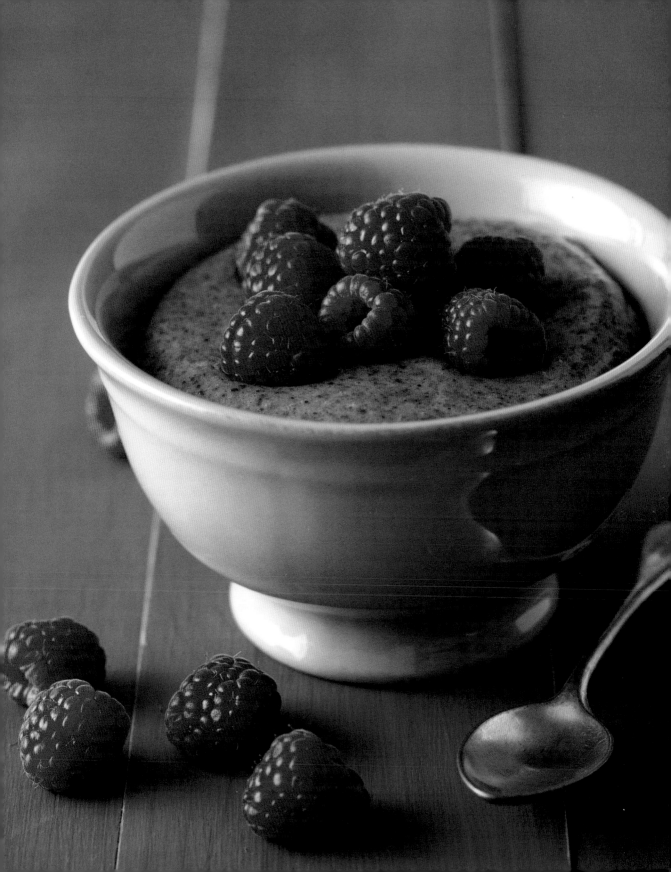

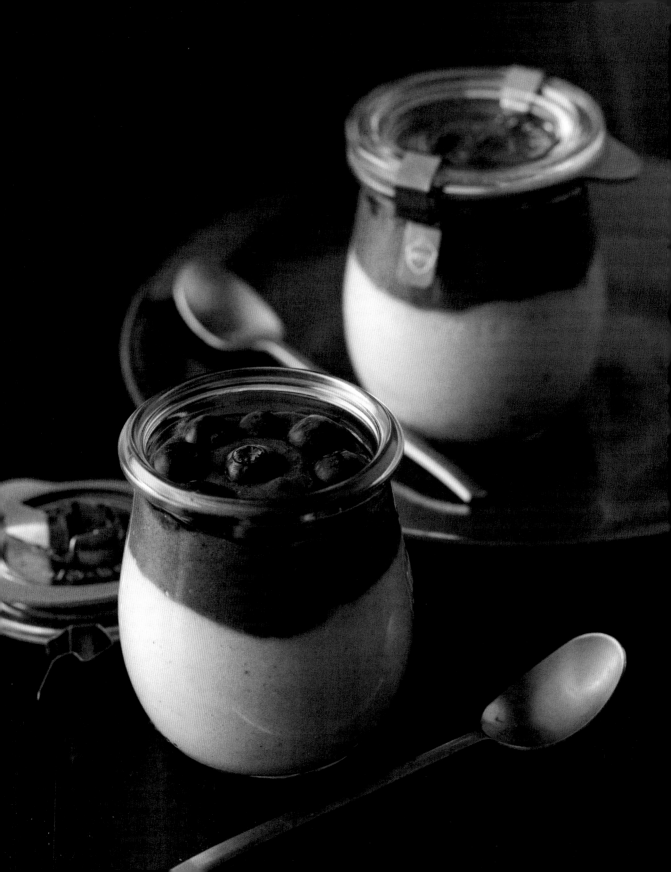

Harmony:
BANANA BERRY NICE CREAM

MAKES 4 SERVINGS (SERVING SIZE: ¾ CUP)

V *Vegan*   **GF** *Gluten-free*

It's hard to say no to a nice bowl of ice cream after dinner, especially if it's a balanced blend of just pure, whole ingredients instead of a traditional added-sugar-packed pint. A cup of raspberries has 8 grams of fiber—making them one of the most fiberlicious fruits around! The berrier the merrier!

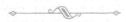

Blend the frozen bananas until semi-smooth in a high-powered blender. Spoon the bananas into a small bowl or jar. Place the berries and, if using, the pomegranate powder in the blender and blend until creamy. Layer the berries on top of the banana mixture. Dress with the topping, if desired.

3 small frozen bananas

1 cup frozen raspberries

1 cup frozen blueberries

1 cup frozen strawberries

1 tablespoon pomegranate Powerfood Powder (optional)

OPTIONAL TOPPING

1 tablespoon berries of your choice

MEAL MATH per serving						
calories	fat	sodium	carbs	fiber	sugar	protein
120	0.5g	0mg	30g	6g	16g	2g

Do-It-Yourself Ingredients

When you're cooking from scratch in your own kitchen, you get to call all the shots—that means you own the power of controlling whatever is going into your food. In terms of cost, most of the time it's actually cheaper to make these kitchen staples yourself. These recipes will give you an easy-to-follow play-by-play on how to do it your way.

VEGAN YOGURT

MAKES 4 SERVINGS (SERVING SIZE: ¼ CUP)

V Vegan   **GF** Gluten-free

When it comes to all the digestive health bonuses in yogurt, there's plenty to brag about. You can make my easy homemade and dairy-free version of this nutritious powerfood—and it's actually higher in fiber, lower in sugar, and lacking all the extra ingredients you might find in most vegan store-bought varieties! This recipe will supply your breakfast soups with a thick, creamy texture and natural sweetness.

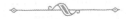

Place the milk, chia seeds, vanilla, syrup, cinnamon, and probiotic powder in a high-powered blender and blend for 1 minute. Chill in a sealed container for at least 20 minutes before using. Or, if using ground chia or ground flaxseed, simply combine all ingredients, stir well, and let chill for 20 minutes.

1 cup unsweetened plant-based milk (see page 139)

2 tablespoons whole or ground chia seeds or flaxseeds

1 teaspoon pure vanilla extract

1 tablespoon pure maple syrup

½ teaspoon Ceylon cinnamon

4 doses probiotic powder*

*Find at a health food store or online. Look for powders containing the strains *Lactobacillus* and *Bifidobacterium*. Make sure the label reads "live and active cultures" with colony-forming units in the billions. And store refrigerated in an airtight container away from heat and moisture.

Power Up!

ADD TO RECIPE:

¼ teaspoon ground nutmeg

MEAL MATH per serving						
calories	fat	sodium	carbs	fiber	sugar	protein
60	3g	70mg	5g	3g	3g	2g

SPICED BUCKWHEAT GRANOLA

MAKES 64 SERVINGS (SERVING SIZE: 1 TABLESPOON)

V Vegan   **GF** Gluten-free

If you pay attention to labels, most store-bought varieties of this favorite breakfast food are basically cookie crumbs costumed as healthful granola. Instead, fill yourself up with a bowl that comes naturally gluten-free and boasts vitamin B–rich buckwheat groats, anti-inflammatory-packed spices, and tons of fiber and healthful fats. A little sweet, slightly spicy, and completely loaded with good-for-you ingredients—this is the way I like my granola in the morning.

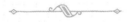

2 cups buckwheat groats

1½ cups mixed seeds and nuts (I like sliced almonds)

1 cup unsweetened coconut flakes

1 teaspoon Ceylon cinnamon

1 teaspoon ground ginger

2 teaspoons granulated orange peel

2 tablespoons coconut oil

2 tablespoons pure maple syrup

1 ripe banana, mashed (optional)

Preheat the oven to 350° F.

In a medium bowl, stir the buckwheat groats together with the seeds and nuts, coconut flakes, cinnamon, ginger, and orange peel. Add the coconut oil, maple syrup, and, if using, the mashed banana to the groats mixture; stir until evenly coated. Line a baking sheet with parchment paper, spread the groats mixture evenly on it, and bake for 20 to 30 minutes, stirring once halfway through, until fragrant and golden. Let cool before storing.

MEAL MATH per serving						
calories	fat	sodium	carbs	fiber	sugar	protein
40	2g	0mg	1g	<1g	<1g	1g

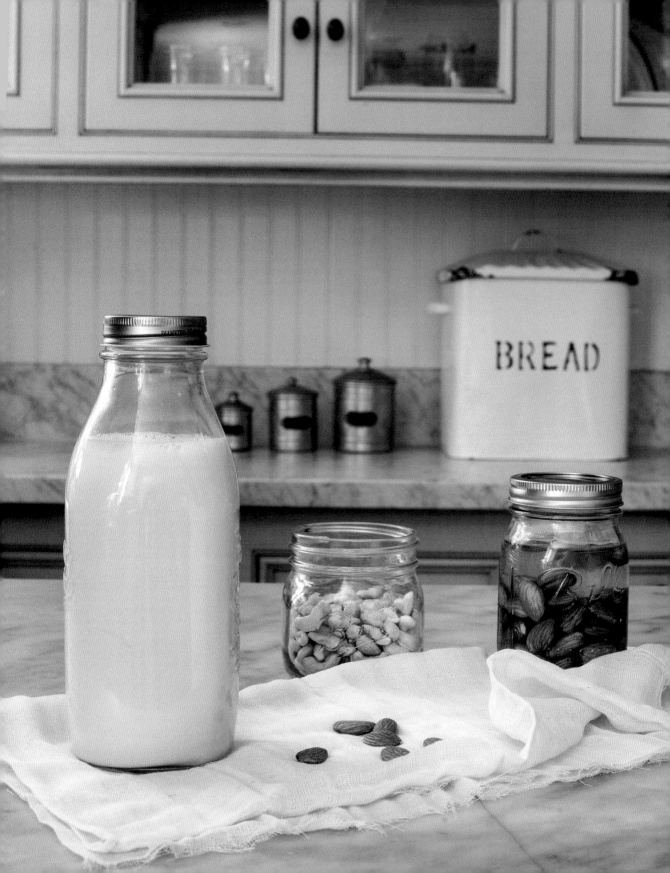

PLANT-BASED MILK

MAKES 4 CUPS (SERVING SIZE: 1 CUP)

V Vegan **GF** Gluten-free

If you've never tasted the homemade version of this kitchen staple, you're missing out! Nothing in the store delivers the same fresh quality and rich taste (I try to make this a few times a month). Even better, you can customize this recipe with different optional add-ins so the flavor possibilities are truly infinite! Don't want to throw out the pulp afterward? I don't blame you—use the leftover pulp in breakfast soups, baked goods, or oatmeal for additional plant-based power perks.

2 cups raw almonds, cashews, or other nut

6 cups filtered water

½ teaspoon Ceylon cinnamon (optional)

1 teaspoon pure vanilla extract (optional)

Pinch of Himalayan or sea salt, to enhance flavor (optional)

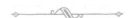

Place the nuts in a bowl and soak overnight in filtered water until they feel slightly squishy. Rinse the nuts thoroughly with cold running water, then drain. Place them in a high-powered blender along with the 6 cups filtered water and any optional ingredients you're using. Blend on high speed for 1 to 2 minutes, until frothy. Strain through a cheesecloth or nut-milk bag, squeezing to extract as much as possible. Store the plant milk in a sealed glass container in the fridge for up to 3 days.

MEAL MATH per serving; approximate due to straining process						
calories	fat	sodium	carbs	fiber	sugar	protein
5	0g	5mg	0g	0g	0g	0g

BEANS

1 POUND DRY BEANS = ABOUT 5 CUPS COOKED

V *Vegan*   GF *Gluten-free*

1 pound dry beans
Filtered water

FLAVOR EXTRAS
1 whole onion
4 garlic cloves
2 bay leaves
Fresh ginger
Fresh fennel
Himalayan or sea salt
Freshly ground black pepper
Olive oil

Prepared beans are a great bargain—but did you know home-cooked beans are about 80 percent cheaper? Plus, you can flavor them however you like and forgo large amounts of excess sodium. Follow my easy DIY steps for an abundance of fresh beans you can throw into your soups, use as healthful protein toppers, or just enjoy as a snack. Feel free to double the amount and freeze leftovers for a convenient, anytime supply.

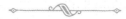

Clean: Rinse beans and discard the rinse water.

Soak: Soak the beans for 4 to 6 hours (I usually soak overnight for convenience) in a pot or bowl filled with filtered water.

Rinse: Strain the beans and rinse them with very cold filtered water. This can help remove some of the gas-producing enzymes that occur naturally in beans.

Add water: Put the beans into a large pot and cover with about 2 inches of fresh filtered water.

Flavor: Toss in some flavor! I like to add onion, garlic, bay leaves, and a few slices of fresh ginger or fennel (both have reducing properties).

Cook: Bring to a boil over medium-high heat and skim off any foam. Reduce to a simmer with the lid off for the remaining cooking time. The one exception is kidney beans, which must be boiled for 10 minutes first and then simmered.

Cooking Times:

Black, cannellini, and azuki: 45–60 minutes

Kidney, navy, and pinto: 1–1½ hours

Garbanzo: 1½–2½ hours

You'll know they're done when the beans are tender and can be easily pierced or mashed.

Season: Season to taste with salt and pepper. Finish with a drizzle of olive oil.

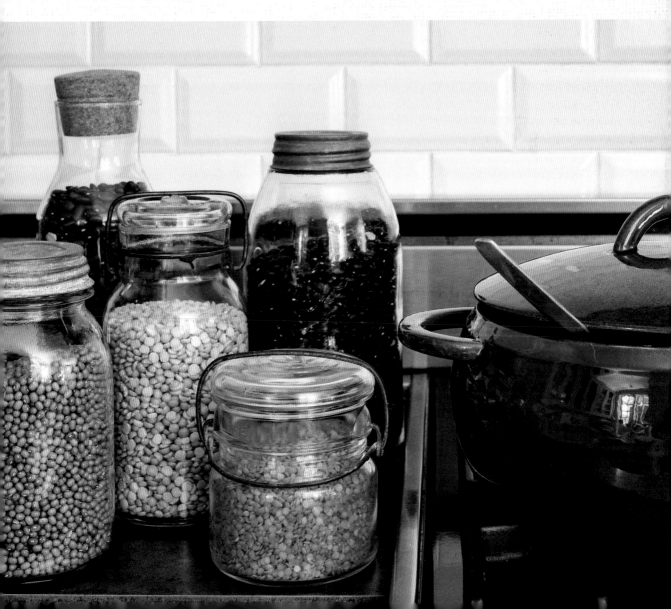

SIMPLE LOW-AND-SLOW BONE BROTH

GF *Gluten-free*

3 to 4 pounds grass-fed beef bones or organic chicken bones

3 tablespoons apple cider vinegar

Filtered water

2 large onions (skins on), cut in half

3 carrots, cut into large pieces

3 stalks celery, cut into large pieces

6 cloves garlic

Small bundle of fresh parsley

Small bundle of thyme

2 bay leaves

2 teaspoons whole black peppercorns

Himalayan or sea salt

ADD-INS FOR EXTRA CREDIT (AND EXTRA NUTRIENTS!)

Fresh ginger, peeled and sliced

Fresh turmeric root, peeled and sliced

Fresh beet, peeled and sliced

Sea vegetables (kombu, nori, wakame)

Herbs (dried or fresh)

Bone broth is being touted as a magic health elixir. While we still don't fully understand the extent of its nutritious wizardry, we do know that cooking the bones with apple cider vinegar may help extract key minerals like calcium, magnesium, and phosphorus— all of which are essential for healthful cellular function. What's more, bone broth contains other elements that may aid in joint, digestive, and immune health, making it go from sounding a little bizarre to totally brilliant. Use this bone broth as a blank canvas to make other more elaborate soups or simply sip as is!

This recipe uses a slow cooker—so you can just throw everything in and forget about it for the day. But you can also do this in a large pot on your stovetop. Make sure the soup stays just below the simmering point.

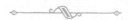

Place the bones in a slow cooker and add the vinegar and enough filtered water to cover the bones by about an inch. Stir in the onion, carrots, celery, garlic, herb bundles, bay leaves, and peppercorns and set the slow cooker on low. Allow to cook for at least 12 hours, and up to 24 hours. Strain and discard the solids. Season with salt to taste.

VEGAN BONE BROTH

V Vegan   **GF** Gluten-free

I know what you're thinking: Hello—how can a bone broth be vegan? And you're absolutely right. This recipe doesn't contain any real bones, but rest assured—the dried seaweed and savory miso paste step up to the plate to deliver an extra-healthful dose of vitamins and minerals. These plant-based ingredients may also improve digestive and immune function and rev up your engine with a revitalizing energy boost.

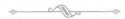

Heat the oil in a large pot over medium heat. Add the celery and leeks and sauté 5 minutes, until softened. Pour in the filtered water. Drain the wakame and add to the pot, along with the beets, garlic, ginger, turmeric, and bay leaf and bring to a boil. Reduce the heat and simmer, covered, for 45 minutes to 2 hours—the flavor will deepen the longer it simmers. Add the miso and parsley and stir until the miso dissolves. Strain the broth and discard the solids. Season with salt and pepper to taste and serve.

2 tablespoons olive oil

2 cups chopped celery

2 leeks, chopped

16 cups filtered water

1 tablespoon dried wakame, reconstituted in a little filtered water

2 golden beets, peeled and chopped

2 garlic cloves

5 or 6 (1-inch) pieces fresh ginger, peeled and sliced

5 or 6 (1-inch) pieces fresh turmeric, peeled and sliced

1 bay leaf

¼ cup organic miso paste of your choice

Handful of fresh parsley leaves

Himalayan or sea salt and freshly ground black pepper

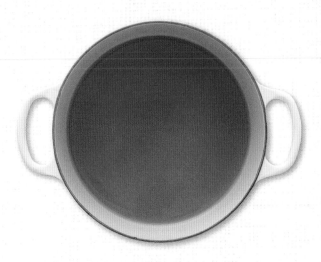

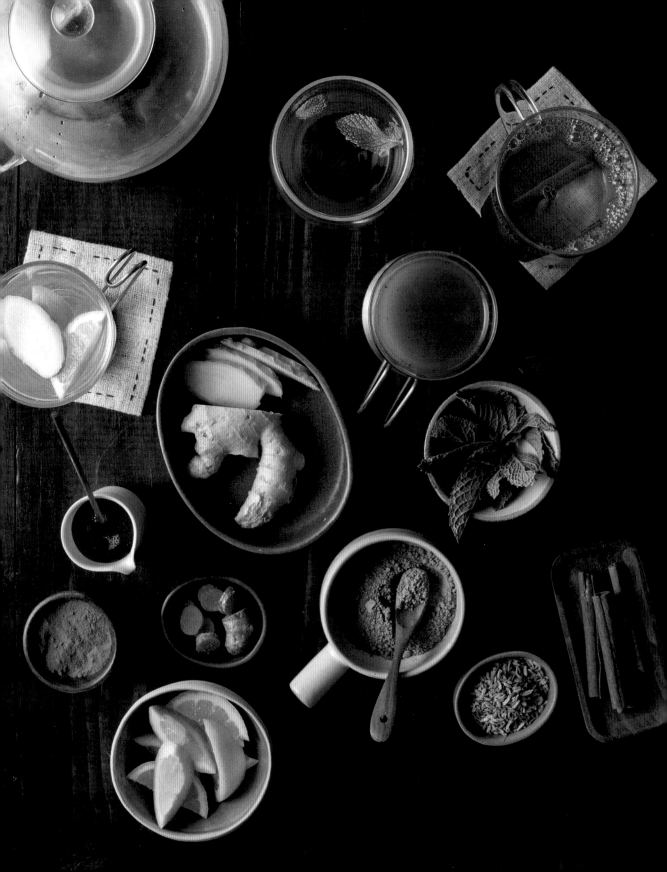

2.

Restart Me in 3

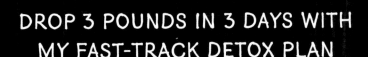

DROP 3 POUNDS IN 3 DAYS WITH MY FAST-TRACK DETOX PLAN

Let's do this! Commit to souping for 3 days (it's only 72 hours) and you'll have more energy and lose up to 3 pounds in the process. More importantly, you'll detox without deprivation. I see it happen all the time with my clients, and I love seeing the sense of empowerment they get after just 3 days on my souping Restart Plan.

For this short period of time, you'll follow a strict menu—but don't worry, you'll get loads of filling, body-cleansing food to meet all of your nutritional requirements. It's commitment time—absolutely no wavering! That means no mindless snacking or extras. If you want to see results, you must go all in.

n for Your 3-Day Restart:

ly from the recommended soups in this chapter. And make the rec-
ook. No extras!

fast every morning. No skipping for any reason!

3. Have a snack every afternoon. It's mandatory—trust me.

4. Ditch coffee and alcohol for the next 3 days. Instead, start your day with my A.M. riser and end it with the P.M. relaxer.

That's it! I've kept it really simple, so there's no room for error.

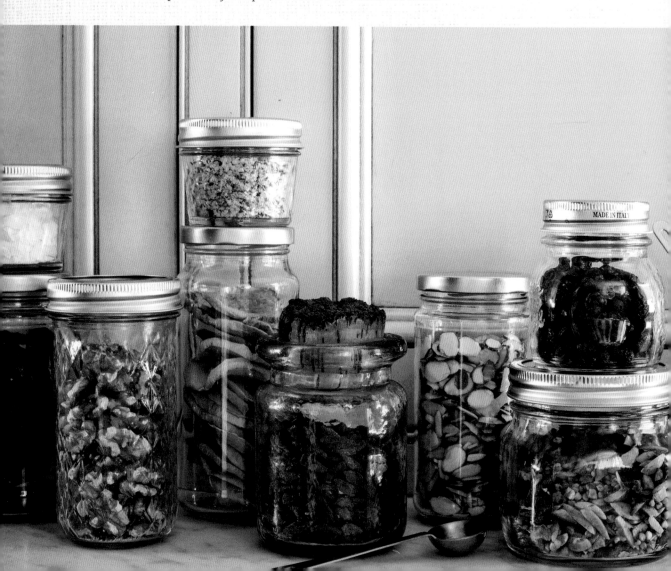

Snacks
Pg. 103 Succulent berry (purple potion)
Pg. 106 Raspberry Kefir (use yogurt)

Your at-a-Glance Meal Guide

Below are my suggestions of what to eat for the next 3 days.

You'll notice that all the recipes in the Restart are vegan. This plant-based approach may be new to you, but it's only for the next few days. I find it's the easiest way to get your fill of critical antioxidants and detoxifying fiber from the big increase of fruits, vegetables, and plant-based proteins. My hope is that after the 3 days are up, you'll feel inspired to continue on a more plant-focused path.

Feel free to swap in any of the other vegan souping options on pages 26–114. I've repeated some of the soups here for simplicity so you can get a few meals out of one batch. Remember to top each bowl with one of my Power Ups to make it soup-erior. Additionally, have 1 cup of any of my detoxifying Freebie Soups if you find yourself wanting a little something extra.

DAY 1

A.M. riser

breakfast
Radiance:
Carrot Cake (page 30)

lunch ½ recipe
Debloat Me:
Green Pea, Asparagus, and Parsley (page 64)

afternoon snack
Invigorate Me:
Spanish Red Pepper (page 101)

dinner
Sustain Me:
Veg-Loaded Lentil (page 68)
4 Real Food whole life recipe

P.M. relaxer

freebie soup of your choice
Optional

ST zucchini soup

DAY 2

A.M. riser

breakfast
Balance Me:
Berries and Greens (page 42)

lunch ½ recipe
Squash Soirée:
Garden-Green Minestrone (page 72)

afternoon snack
Soothe Me:
Blueberry Spice (page 105)

dinner
Debloat Me:
Green Pea, Asparagus, and Parsley (page 64)

P.M. relaxer

freebie soup of your choice
Optional
½ rec.
Immunity
Revive recipe
immunity

DAY 3

A.M. riser

breakfast
Apple-Teeny:
Apple Strawberry (page 51)

lunch
Sustain Me:
Veg-Loaded Lentil (page 68)

afternoon snack
Endless Summer:
Cucumber Avocado (page 102)

dinner Smoky Black Bean
Fulfill Me:
Hearty Black Bean (page 83)
½ recipe

P.M. relaxer

freebie soup of your choice
Optional

Breakfast

As a mother of four, I understand what it means to be rushed in the morning! But I always think of A.M. as standing for **a**bsolutely **m**andatory—no matter how early, late, or insane my morning is, I never miss breakfast, and I don't want you to, either. So here's the plan:

Start with the A.M. riser (see page 150). This elixir will give you a metabolic bump and a hit of antioxidants—while also delivering a gentle caffeine fix.

Now Enjoy a Restart Me Smoothie Bowl. If you're looking to detox and drop pounds, you need a *real*, fiberized cleanse in the morning—not just any old smoothie. For the next 3 days, choose from one of these fiber-tox souper-bowls:

- Radiance: Carrot Cake (page 30)

- Balance Me: Berries and Greens (page 42)

- Apple-Teeny: Apple Strawberry (page 51)

Lunch and Dinner

Your midday and evening soups are interchangeable—and all of the recipes make multiple batches, so you'll have ready-made meals in the fridge. You can eat the same soup every day for lunch and dinner, or try a different soup each time; extras can also be frozen.

Have one of the following savory soups:

- Debloat Me: Green Pea, Asparagus, and Parsley (page 64)

- Sustain Me: Veg-Loaded Lentil (page 68)

- Squash Soirée: Garden-Green Minestrone (page 72)

- Fulfill Me: Hearty Black Bean (page 83)

Afternoon Snack

As with breakfast, your P.M. snack is positively **m**andatory—there are just too many hours between lunch and dinner. If you skip your afternoon snack, you'll suffer one of the three C's:

Crashing (no energy!)

Cravings ("*Mmm*, I could really go for some pretzels," which will lead to . . .)

Cheating (vending machine raid!)

So here's the deal. Eat a mandatory P.M. snack soup:

- Invigorate Me: Spanish Red Pepper (page 101)
- Soothe Me: Blueberry Spice (page 105)
- Endless Summer: Cucumber Avocado (page 102)

After Dinner

Wind down with my P.M. relaxer (see page 150). To get your body ready for a good night's sleep (adequate rest is essential for weight loss!), put away the hard stuff. Those are calories you don't need, and this plan is supposed to be about detoxing! Instead, cozy up with a cup of my P.M. relaxer tea—it's a natural debloater and aids digestion. Keep this habit going to rock a flat tummy.

A.M. RISER

MAKES 1 DRINK

Stir ½ teaspoon matcha powder into 1 cup hot water and add a squeeze of fresh lemon, lime, or orange juice. Stir the tea as you drink—otherwise the matcha will sink to the bottom of the mug.

If matcha's not your thing, try one of these options. Find whatever suits you best and consider it your A.M. riser from here on out:

- Combine 1 cup hot green tea with one ½-inch slice peeled fresh ginger (just let it steep in the liquid). Add a squeeze of lemon and a cinnamon stick.

- Want a caffeine-free option? Combine 1 cup hot water with one ½-inch slice peeled fresh ginger (steeped in the water), a squeeze of lemon, and a cinnamon stick.

- Mix ¼ teaspoon ground turmeric (or one ½-inch piece peeled fresh turmeric root), ½ teaspoon raw honey, and the juice of ½ lemon into a mug of warm water. Add a dash of cinnamon (optional). Stir to keep the turmeric from settling on the bottom.

P.M. RELAXER

MAKES 1 DRINK

Place 1 chamomile tea bag in 1 cup hot water. Add 3 to 5 fresh mint leaves, ½ teaspoon fennel seeds, and two ½-inch slices peeled fresh ginger, allow to steep for 5 minutes before sipping.

Quick Questions

What if I get hungry after dinner?

Go ahead and have 1 cup of any of the Freebie Soups starting on page 116.

What if I fall off the diet for a meal? Should I just add another day, or do I have to start over?

Add another day.

I finished the 3-Day Restart but didn't lose as much weight as I wanted to. Should I do it again?

No, go straight to the next chapter. I've found that the Restart yields, on average, a 3-pound loss. But everyone is different. Be proud of your success! The 24-day plan that follows is designed to keep fast-tracking your weight loss—so continue the journey.

Okay, I did it and lost weight! Now what?

Now you move on to the next souping stage: The 24-Day Transformation. It's the quick and easy way to continue shedding pounds and reaping major health benefits. And I'll teach you simple yet enormously effective nutritional principles that you'll stick to for life. Just turn to the next chapter to get started.

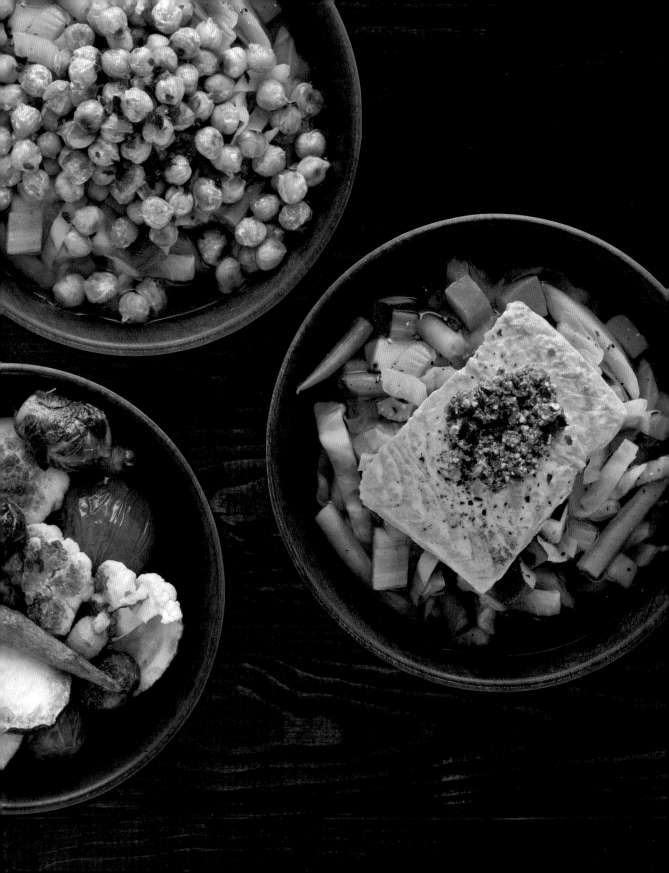

3.

Transform Me in 24

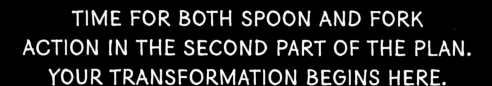

TIME FOR BOTH SPOON AND FORK ACTION IN THE SECOND PART OF THE PLAN. YOUR TRANSFORMATION BEGINS HERE.

Now that you've completed your 3-Day Restart, you should already look and feel lighter—and be motivated to drop even more weight during the next few weeks.

In addition to souping—keep that spoon handy!— I'll show you how to mix in plated meals as a transition to a realistic and sustainable lifestyle. I'm also opening up your options to include recipes that offer something for everyone—the vegan, vegetarian, pescetarian, meat eater, and gluten-free devotee.

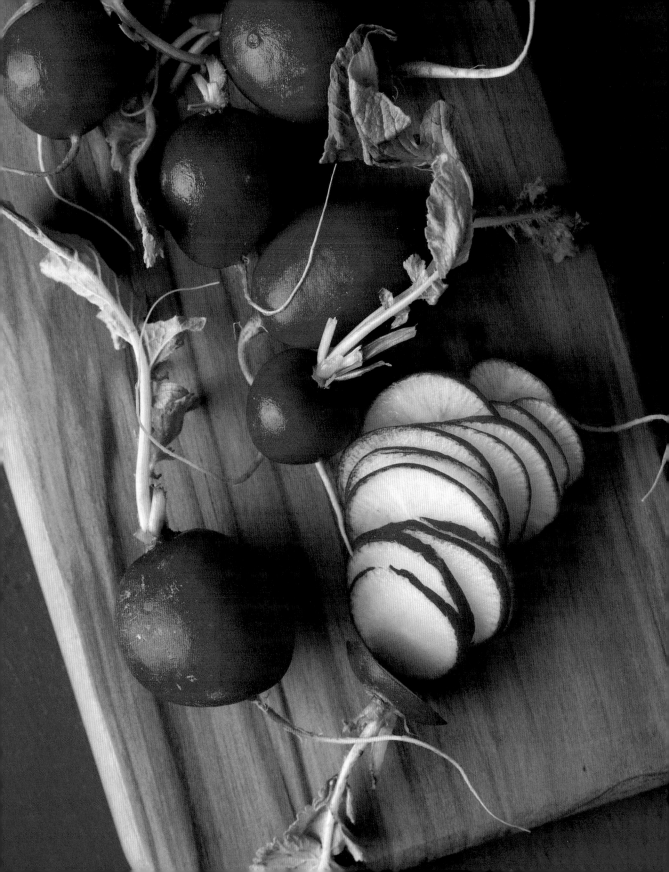

Why 24 days? You may have heard that it takes 21 days to form a habit—which is what a lot of other diets are based on. But I've found in my personal practice that building a few extra days into this part of the plan solidifies people's long-term commitment and ensures success better than a strictly 3-week plan.

Now here's the game plan:

1. **Soup at least once a day.** It's a must for either lunch or dinner. Extra credit for breaking out a bowl for breakfast or snack time, too.

2. **Select *only* from the soups in Chapter 1 or the plated meals at the end of this chapter.** If you loved the meals from the 3-Day Restart, feel free to make them again, but you now have a wider range of soups to choose from—plus the plated meals you'll find starting on page 173. You can sample something new every day or make a big batch of a lunch or dinner soup and eat it all week—but no wandering!

3. **Keep snacking every afternoon.** You can also have an after-dinner treat but only if you feel the need.

4. **Add in coffee but not alcohol.** You can have 1 cup of organic coffee each day if you like but not in place of the A.M. riser. And no alcohol for the next 24 days.

5. **Sip your A.M. riser and P.M. relaxer daily.**

6. **Learn "the Rules."** Understanding the logic behind my guidelines—which I'll get to shortly—will make it easier to DIY and maintain your success once you graduate from the plan. Consider the next 24 days training for years to come.

7. **Keep it real.** Real foods get real results. Stick to natural wholesome foods and cut out manufactured messes that sound like science experiments. But remember, no matter how clean you eat, it's a myth that clean eating = all you can eat (see page 239 for more).

Simple, right? From my experience, straightforward and realistic works best.
Now let's dig in.

Your 1-Week Meal-Planning Calendar

To make the next 3 weeks even easier, I've put together a sample 7-day meal calendar that includes both soups and plated meals. As with the Restart, you don't need to follow this exact schedule. Feel free to mix and match dishes, depending on your tastes, and use this as a guide to map out your day. Just remember to soup at either lunch or dinner. If you're wanting a little something more or are just craving an extra dose of detox, have any of the Freebie Soups (see pages 116–117).

Print out a copy of this chart! You can find it on my website, www.bellernutritional institute.com.

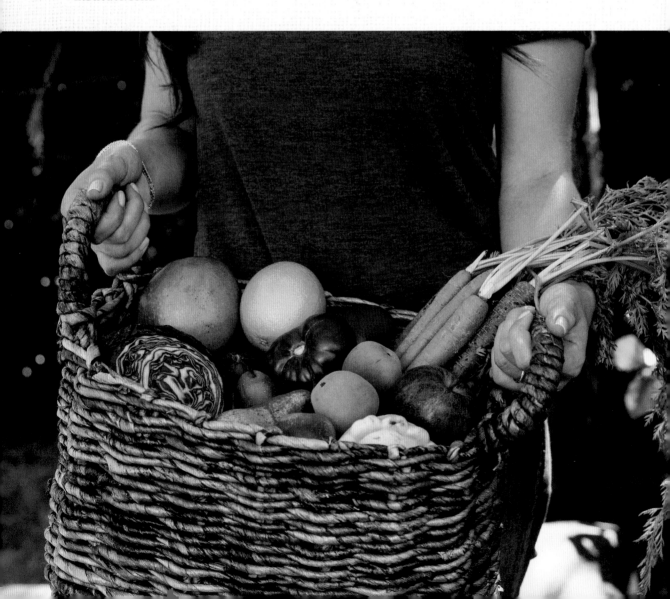

Mon	Tue	Wed	Thurs	Fri	Sat	
A.M. riser	**A.M. riser**	**A.M. riser**	**A.M. riser**	**A.M. riser**	**A.M. riser**	
breakfast *The Beller Basic:* Simple Greens (page 33)	**breakfast** CinSational Quinoa (page 179)	**breakfast** *Inner Child:* Peanut Butter and Jelly (page 41)	**breakfast** *Happy Gut:* Kefir Pour and Go (page 52)	**breakfast** Apple with Appeal Oatmeal (page 178)	**breakfast** *Detoxi-Pie Me:* Creamy Almond Peach Pie (page 37)	breakfast *Glowing Green:* Sweet Ginger Kale (page 45)
lunch Chickpea Salad (page 184)	**lunch** *Ignite Me:* Tuscan-Style White Beans (page 63)	**lunch** Mixed salad + Zesty Edamame— (page 200) + ¼ avocado	**lunch** *Strengthen Me:* Savory Split Pea (page 80), + Simple Roasted Veg (page 193)	**lunch** Mixed salad + Egg White-ish Salad (page 202)	**lunch** *Zen-Sational:* Mung Bean (page 79)	**lunch** Mediterranean Bowl (page 181)
afternoon snack 1 medium apple with 1 egg	**afternoon snack** *Blush:* Raspberry Kefir (page 106)	**afternoon snack** peanuts + cacao nibs + coconut flakes (page 167)	**afternoon snack** *Purple Potion:* Succulent Berry (page 103)	**afternoon snack** 1 cup strawberries + 11 cashews (see pages 168–169)	**afternoon snack** ½ cup Spiced Chickpeas (page 201)	**afternoon snack** ¼ cup Basic Hummus (page 207) + 1 cup celery sticks
dinner *Ignite Me:* Tuscan-Style White Beans (page 63)	**dinner** Simple Sautéed Spinach (page 189) + Speedy Broiled Salmon (page 196) + 1 tsp pine nuts	**dinner** *Strengthen Me:* Split Pea (page 80) + Simple Roasted Veg (page 193)	**dinner** Fish in a Packet (page 186)	**dinner** *Zen-Sational:* Mung Bean (page 79)	**dinner** *Greeeeen 5:* Greens, Beans, and Things (page 88)	**dinner** *Comfort Me:* Creamy Tomato (page 67)
after dinner (optional) Almond-stuffed Medjool date (page 167)	**after dinner (optional)** ½ ounce (3 small squares) dark chocolate + 20 pistachios	**after dinner (optional)** *Harmony:* Banana Berry Nice Cream (page 133)	**after dinner (optional)** 20 frozen grapes	**after dinner (optional)** *Clarity:* Berry Rich (page 126)	**after dinner (optional)** 1 Greek Yogurt Frozen Pop (page 215) + 11 cashews	**after dinner (optional)** *Crave Me:* A Date with Chocolate (page 130)
P.M. relaxer	**P.M. relaxer**	**P.M. relaxer**	**P.M. relaxer**	**P.M. relaxer**	**P.M. relaxer**	**P.M. relaxer**
freebie soup	freebie soup	freebie soup	freebie soup	freebie soup	freebie soup	freebie soup

The Rule of 3: How to Build a Meal

My goal is to make nutrition as uncomplicated as possible, which is why I have mapped out exactly what you need to eat for the next 24 days. But I also want to let you in on the principles of how I put together each meal and snack in this plan—because you'll be using them once you reach the Maintenance phase. Also, you may need to refer to these rules during the 24-Day Transformation if you can't have one of my approved recipes when you're out and about (life happens, I get it!). I've pared down all the complex nutrition info so that whether you're souping or plating, you just have to follow my essential rules. You don't need to memorize them all right now, but getting the hang of the general concepts will make cooking and eating out on your own after the 24 days that much more intuitive.

The Rule of 3: Breakfast

1. Fiber Up: Get at least 10 grams of fiber. Front-loading with an A.M. "fiber fix" fast-tracks you to your daily goal of 30 to 35 grams.
   Fiber is key for:

> *Daily detox*
> *Digestive health*
> *Heart health*
> *Steady energy*
> *Cancer prevention*
> *Blood sugar regulation*

Note: Grains are *not* allowed after breakfast during the 24-Day Transformation.

2. Plant 1: Include at least 1 serving of produce. I'm talking about whole fruits and veggies, not just the juice. And sugary dried cranberries in a protein bar don't count!

3. Eye Cals: Limit this meal to 350 "real food" calories—max. Pay attention to calories to avoid going overboard on clean foods that promise you the moon (such a common pitfall!). You'll only wind up with a full-moon-shaped figure.

EXTRA CREDIT: POWER UP!

Every recipe in this book is designed to ensure you get an optimal range of vitamins and minerals. But I want you to upgrade and amp up the nutrition even more by adding these superstars to your meals. Check out pages 56–59.

Note: You may add in more protein, if you're doing some major workouts or just feel you need a little more. Think: 1 tablespoon protein powder or hemp seeds or 2 organic egg whites. Just watch that clean food 350-calorie limit!

The Rule of 3: Lunch and Dinner

1. Veg Out: Load up on about 2 cups of low-starch veggies. They deliver antioxidants, help detox your system, and fill you up for very few calories—making the weight fall off in a powerful way. Enjoy your veggies any way you like them: in a soup or salad, raw, roasted or sautéed in a tiny bit of high-quality oil.

Low-starch vegetables—eat all you want!

alfalfa sprouts	cauliflower	horseradish	romaine
artichoke	celery	jicama	rutabaga
arugula	chard	kale	shallot
asparagus	chives	kohlrabi	spinach
bamboo shoots	collard greens	leeks	sprouts
bean sprouts	cucumber	lettuce	summer squash
beets*	daikon radish	mushrooms	Swiss chard
bell peppers	eggplant	okra	tomato*
bok choy	endive	onions	turnip greens
broccoli	escarole	peppers (all varieties)	turnips
broccoli sprouts	fennel	radicchio	water chestnuts
Brussels sprouts	green beans	radish	watercress
cabbage	green onion	rhubarb	zucchini
carrots*			

Beets, carrots, and tomatoes are higher in sugar than other veg, so don't go overboard.

Starchy vegetables to avoid during the 24 days: butternut squash, corn, potatoes, pumpkins, and yams.

2. Go Pro: Include 1 serving of protein. No matter what your protein preferences are (vegan, vegetarian, or other), you need it to boost your immunity, keep your muscles strong, provide long-lasting energy, and make your meal more satisfying.

What does 1 serving of protein look like?
150 TO 200 CALORIES per serving

Beans and legumes	¾ cup, cooked
Peas	1½ cups, cooked
Organic sprouted tofu, edamame, tempeh	1 cup, cooked
Seafood (low mercury, omega-3 rich)	4 ounces (about the size of your computer's mouse), cooked
Organic eggs	2 whole large eggs OR 1 whole large egg, plus 2 whites OR 6 egg whites
Organic poultry or grass-fed beef	4 ounces, cooked
Organic plain 2% Greek yogurt or kefir	1 cup

3. Fatten Up: Add 1 to 2 servings of fat. Good-for-you fats help you feel fuller longer and allow your body to absorb more vitamins, minerals, and cancer-fighting phytonutrients. Select any you like from this list. And feel free to mix it up. For example, you could have two servings of oil (1 tablespoon)—or have one serving of oil (½ tablespoon) + one serving of avocado (¼ fruit).

50 TO 60 CALORIES per serving

High-quality oils and spreads:
  olive oil
  coconut oil
  avocado oil
  walnut oil
  ghee [occasional]
  tahini
	½ tablespoon (1½ teaspoons)

Nuts and seeds:
  almonds
  walnuts
  pine nuts
  shelled pistachios
  chia seeds
  sunflower seeds
  pumpkin seeds
  sesame seeds
	1 tablespoon

Fruit:
  avocado
  guacamole
	¼ fruit
	2 tablespoons

Other:
  cashew crème (see page 206)
  pesto (see pages 203–204)
  dressings (see pages 210–211)
	1 tablespoon

EXTRA CREDIT: POWER UP!

Remember to boost your meals even more by adding these healthful superstars to your meal. And they're virtually calorie-free, so help yourself! For even more ideas, see pages 92–96.

- Spices, such as turmeric, cinnamon, ginger, and garlic
- Fresh or dried herbs, like parsley, basil, and cilantro
- Fresh or granulated orange, lemon, or lime zest
- Superplants, such as horseradish, broccoli sprouts, and sauerkraut

LUNCH AND DINNER
3-STEP MEAL BUILDING

1. *VEG OUT*
START WITH ABOUT 2 CUPS OF LOW-STARCH VEGGIES:

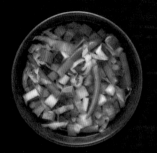

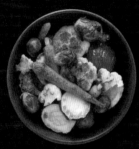

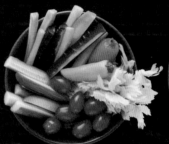

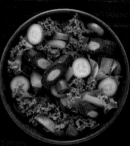

A VEG-LOADED
SOUP

ROASTED/SAUTÉED

RAW

SALAD

2. *GO PRO*
INCLUDE ONE SERVING OF PROTEIN:

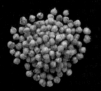

¾ CUP BEANS OR LEGUMES*

1 CUP ORGANIC TOFU OR EDAMAME*

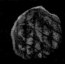

4 OUNCES LOW-
MERCURY FISH

2 WHOLE EGGS

4 OUNCES
POULTRY

4 OUNCES
GRASS-FED BEEF

*VEGAN OPTIONS

3. *FATTEN UP*
ADD 1 TO 2 SERVINGS OF FAT:

  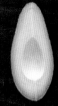

½ TABLESPOON OIL | 1 TABLESPOON NUTS | ¼ AVOCADO

½ TABLESPOON TAHINI | 1 TABLESPOON SEEDS | 1 TABLESPOON CASHEW CRÈME (PAGE 206) OR PESTO (PAGES 203 AND 204) | 1 TABLESPOON NATURAL DRESSING (SEE PAGES 210–212)

CHIA SEEDS | SESAME SEEDS

EXTRA CREDIT: POWER UP!

AMP UP NUTRITION AND FLAVOR WITH MY FAVORITE POWER UPS

  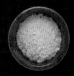 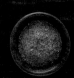

BROCCOLI SPROUTS | FRESH HERBS | NUTRITIONAL YEAST | SAUERKRAUT | SPICE BLEND

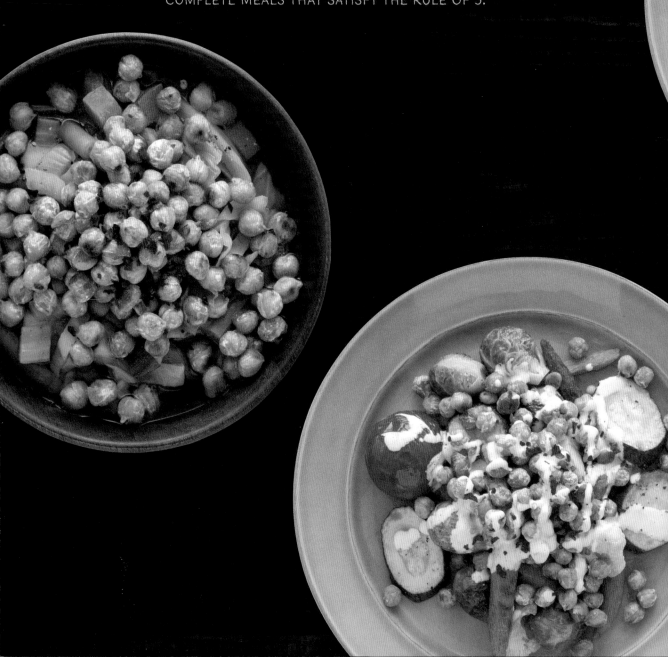

You're done!

HERE ARE SOME EXAMPLES OF VEGAN AND NONVEGAN
COMPLETE MEALS THAT SATISFY THE RULE OF 3.

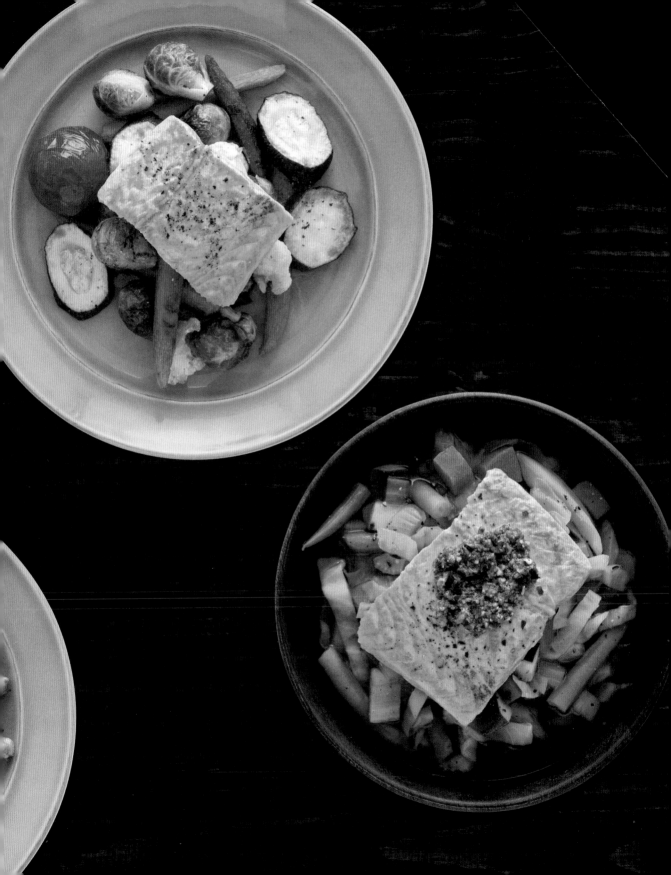

ur Afternoon Snack

an afternoon snack—and if you pass it up, I guarantee that you'll over-
hat to keep in mind:

1. Go Low: Limit it to 150 to 175 calories. Less is fine, but don't go above.

2. Be Real: Keep it clean. Stick to high-quality ingredients you can recognize.

3. Opt Out: Skip the grains and cheese (for now).

SNACK OPTIONS:

Have one of the Snack Time soups (see pages 99–121).

Enjoy any of the Freebie Soups (see pages 116–117).

Have ½ cup of the Spiced Chickpeas on page 201.

Mix and match any of the proteins listed next and the fruits and nuts on pages
168–169. Just keep everything within the 150 to 175 calorie limit!

Proteins
½ cup organic plain 2% Greek yogurt (85 calories)
½ cup shelled organic edamame (94 calories)
½ cup garbanzo beans (134 calories)
1 organic large egg (70 calories)
¼ cup hummus (170 calories)

MIXING IT UP!

My clients love snacks—here are more ideas for your snacking pleasure, all 175 calories or less!

2 tablespoons Cashew Crème (page 206) + 1 cup cucumber slices (136 calories)

2 tablespoons Cinnamon Sweet Crème (page 206) + apple slices from ½ medium apple (167 calories)

¾ cup frozen organic edamame sprinkled with 1 teaspoon sesame seeds (156 calories)

40 pistachios (133 calories)

½ ounce (3 small squares) dark chocolate + 20 pistachios (151 calories)

22 almonds soaked in water + fresh slice of lemon (153 calories)

3 halves Medjool date stuffed with 3 almonds each (162 calories)

20 peanuts + 1 tablespoon cacao nibs + 1 tablespoon unsweetened coconut flakes (167 calories)

¼ cup hummus + celery sticks from 1 stalk celery (175 calories)

2 tablespoons sliced almonds + 2 tablespoons freeze-dried blueberries + 2 tablespoons freeze-dried cranberries + 2 tablespoons unsweetened coconut flakes (166 calories)

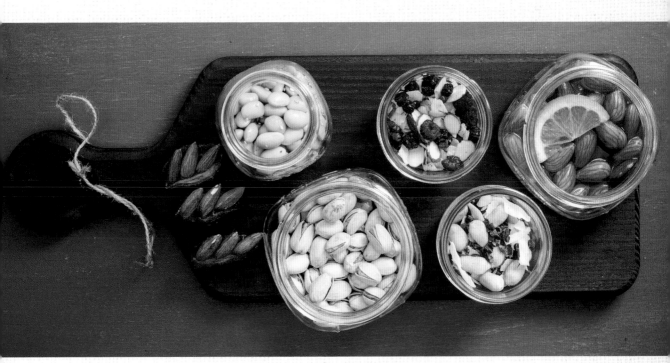

WHOLESOME AND SIMPLE SNACKS

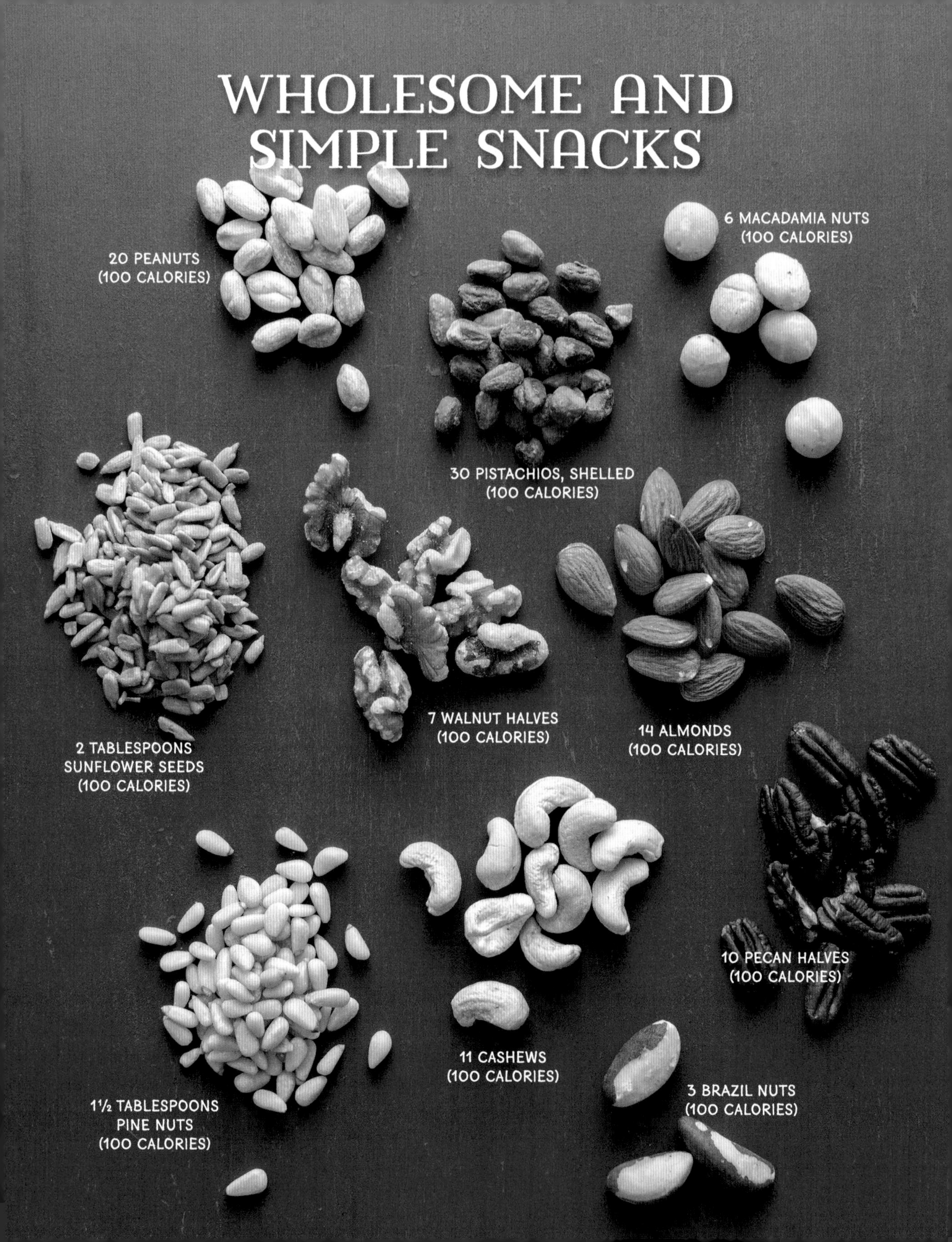

20 PEANUTS
(100 CALORIES)

6 MACADAMIA NUTS
(100 CALORIES)

30 PISTACHIOS, SHELLED
(100 CALORIES)

2 TABLESPOONS
SUNFLOWER SEEDS
(100 CALORIES)

7 WALNUT HALVES
(100 CALORIES)

14 ALMONDS
(100 CALORIES)

10 PECAN HALVES
(100 CALORIES)

1½ TABLESPOONS
PINE NUTS
(100 CALORIES)

11 CASHEWS
(100 CALORIES)

3 BRAZIL NUTS
(100 CALORIES)

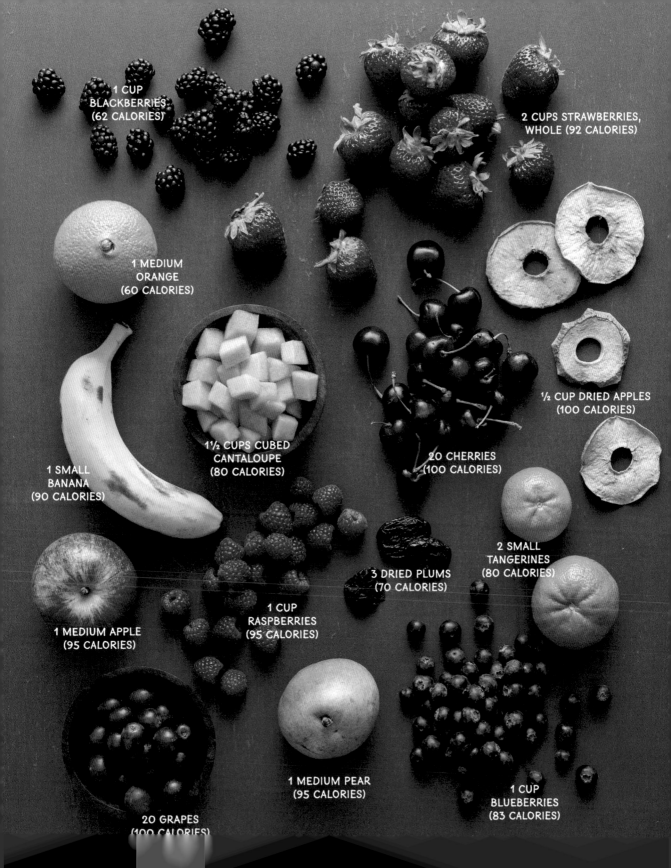

1 CUP
BLACKBERRIES
(62 CALORIES)

2 CUPS STRAWBERRIES,
WHOLE (92 CALORIES)

1 MEDIUM
ORANGE
(60 CALORIES)

½ CUP DRIED APPLES
(100 CALORIES)

1½ CUPS CUBED
CANTALOUPE
(80 CALORIES)

20 CHERRIES
(100 CALORIES)

1 SMALL
BANANA
(90 CALORIES)

2 SMALL
TANGERINES
(80 CALORIES)

3 DRIED PLUMS
(70 CALORIES)

1 MEDIUM APPLE
(95 CALORIES)

1 CUP
RASPBERRIES
(95 CALORIES)

1 MEDIUM PEAR
(95 CALORIES)

1 CUP
BLUEBERRIES
(83 CALORIES)

20 GRAPES
(100 CALORIES)

The Rule of 3: After Dinner

Care for some dessert? Yes, you read that right! In this part of the plan, I'm giving you the option (repeat: *option*) of having an after-dinner treat. You may lose weight a bit faster if you skip it, but I know from experience that some people just want a little something in the evening. Here are the rules for treats:

1. **Check In: Ask yourself if you really need it.**

2. **Go Low: Keep it under 150 calories.**

3. **Be Real: Keep it clean.**

PICK ONE OF THESE REAL-DEAL DESSERTS:

Choose any of the Dessert Soups (see pages 123–133).

Enjoy one of my plated dessert recipes (see pages 214–217):

Have a mixture of:
fruit
pure dark chocolate (3 small squares or ½ ounce of at least 72% cacao)
nuts

Just be sure to keep it under 150 calories. See page 163–169 for caloric values.

Daily Cheat Sheet Checklist

BEFORE BREAKFAST

A.M. riser

BREAKFAST

Fiber Up: at least 10 grams of fiber
Plant 1: at least 1 serving of whole fruits and vegetables
Eye Cals: 350 calories or less
Extra Credit: Power up!

LUNCH/DINNER

Veg Out: about 2 cups of low-starch veggies
Go Pro: 1 serving of protein
Fatten Up: 1 to 2 servings of a healthful fat
Extra Credit: Power up!

P.M. SNACK

Go Low: 150 to 175 calories
Be Real: clean ingredients
Opt Out: no grains or cheeses

DESSERT (OPTIONAL)

Check In: Do you really need it?
Go Low: 150 calories or less
Be Real: clean and natural

AFTER DINNER

P.M. relaxer

FREEBIE SOUP (OPTIONAL)

Quick Questions

What if I have a day when I absolutely can't follow the plan and have to eat on my own?

I get it; I know that you might need to stray from the plan once or twice during the next several weeks. Life happens. Business lunches happen. Birthdays happen. But if you have to fly solo, I want you to do it in the smartest way possible. Do your best to become familiar with the meal building Rule of 3 so you'll feel more confident making the best choices on your own. Refer to the cheat sheet on page 171. Review the rules and spot-check your meal to make sure it satisfies the Rule of 3. Then get right back to the 24-Day Transformation.

If I've had a really active day and want an extra snack, can I have one?

Yes! You can have any of the Freebie Soups on pages 116–117.

What if I get to the end of the 24 days and still need to lose more weight?

Keep going with the Transformation until you hit your goal weight.

Plated Meals — Transformed!

Time to go beyond the bowl. Here you'll find complete breakfast, lunch, dinner, and dessert recipes that all follow my Rule of 3. I've also included mix-and-match protein, veggie, and fat options—so you can put your own plate together when you want more flexibility. Fork in!

Breakfasts

Not in the mood for a smoothie bowl? Change it up with one of the following fiber-insured breakfasts that meet my breakfast Rule of 3.

GREET THE DAY PARFAIT

MAKES 1 SERVING

VO *Vegan option* **GF** *Gluten-free*

Place half of the yogurt in a glass or jar and layer half of the raspberries and chia seeds on top. Repeat, layering remaining yogurt, raspberries, and chia seeds. Top with the buckwheat groats and, if desired, the honey.

1 cup organic plain 2% Greek, goat, or Vegan Yogurt (page 135)

½ cup fresh raspberries

1 tablespoon chia seeds

1 tablespoon buckwheat groats

1 teaspoon raw honey (optional)

Power Up!

TOP WITH OR BLEND IN:

¼ teaspoon raw cacao powder

MEAL MATH per serving							
calories	*fat*	*sodium*	*carbs*	*fiber*	*sugar*	*protein*	
310	10g	120mg	17g	11g	12g	28g	

EGG SQUARES TO GO

MAKES 6 SERVINGS (SERVING SIZE: 2 SQUARES)

GF *Gluten-free*

8 organic large eggs

8 organic egg whites

3 Roma tomatoes, diced

3 cups baby spinach or chopped Swiss chard

½ cup chopped fresh basil or parsley

4 tablespoons chia seeds

½ teaspoon Himalayan or sea salt

¼ teaspoon freshly ground black pepper

Power Up!

ADD TO THE MIXING BOWL:

½ teaspoon turmeric

Preheat the oven to 350°F.

In a medium bowl, whisk the eggs and egg whites. Add the remaining ingredients and mix well to combine.

Line a 9 × 12-inch baking dish with parchment paper and pour in the egg mixture. Bake for 30 to 45 minutes, until the eggs are set. Remove from the oven and set aside to cool for at least 15 minutes before cutting into 12 squares and serving. Leftovers will keep in the fridge for 3 or 4 days—and are great as a pre-workout snack, too!

Add a fruit to meet your A.M. fiber goal: 2 squares + 1 fruit serving

1 cup fresh raspberries or 1 medium apple

MEAL MATH for two squares						
calories	fat	sodium	carbs	fiber	sugar	protein
150	8g	190mg	4g	5g	2g	14g

MEAL MATH for two squares plus fruit						
calories	fat	sodium	carbs	fiber	sugar	protein
214	9g	192mg	18g	11g	7g	15g

PB&J OVERNIGHT OATS

MAKES 1 SERVING

V *Vegan* **GF** *Gluten-free*

In a medium bowl, stir together the oats, milk, chia seeds, raspberries, peanut butter, and honey, if using, and refrigerate overnight.

½ cup gluten-free rolled oats

¾ cup unsweetened plant-based milk (see page 139)

1 tablespoon chia seeds

¾ cup fresh or frozen raspberries or berry of your choice

2 teaspoons peanut butter or other nut butter

1 teaspoon raw honey (optional)

Power Up!

ADD TO YOUR BOWL:

½ teaspoon Ceylon cinnamon

MEAL MATH per serving						
calories	*fat*	*sodium*	*carbs*	*fiber*	*sugar*	*protein*
310	14g	140mg	16g	13g	5g	10g

APPLE WITH APPEAL OATMEAL

MAKES 1 SERVING

 Vegan 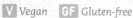 Gluten-free

1 cup cooked gluten-free steel-cut oatmeal

1 small apple, peeled, cored, and chopped

1 tablespoon chia seeds

1 tablespoon hemp seeds

About ¼ unsweetened plant-based milk (optional; see page 139)

Power Up!

ADD TO YOUR BOWL:

½ teaspoon orange zest

Place the oatmeal in a small pot on medium-low heat and stir for 1 minute, adding a little water or plant-based milk if necessary. Transfer the oatmeal to a bowl and stir in the apple, chia seeds, hemp seeds, and the ¼ cup milk, if using (which will give the oatmeal a moister consistency).

MEAL MATH per serving						
calories	fat	sodium	carbs	fiber	sugar	protein
340	12g	10mg	48g	11g	12g	12g

CINSATIONAL QUINOA

MAKES 1 SERVING

V Vegan **GF** Gluten-free

Place the quinoa in a small pot on medium-low heat and stir for 1 minute, adding a little water or plant-based milk if necessary, then transfer to a bowl. In a small saucepan, combine the ½ cup milk, cinnamon, and if using, the vanilla over medium-low heat, about 3 to 5 minutes or until warm. Pour the milk mixture over the quinoa. Gently fold in the blueberries, chia seeds, and the maple syrup, if using.

1 cup cooked quinoa

About ½ cup unsweetened plant-based milk (see page 139)

½ teaspoon Ceylon cinnamon

⅛ teaspoon pure vanilla extract (optional)

½ cup fresh blueberries

1 tablespoon chia seeds

1 teaspoon pure maple syrup (optional)

Power Up!

ADD TO THE SAUCEPAN:

1 teaspoon blueberry Powerfood Powder or Powerfood Powder of your choice (see page 58)

MEAL MATH per serving						
calories	fat	sodium	carbs	fiber	sugar	protein
310	9g	140mg	46g	13g	11g	10g

Lunch and Dinner Plates

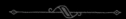

You'll find two different types of plated meals here: First, I'm giving you complete meals that have everything you need in one recipe. Then you'll find mix-and-match meals—which allow you to choose the veg you want and pair it with your protein and healthful fat of your choice.

MEDITERRANEAN BOWL

MAKES 1 SERVING

GF *Gluten-free*

Place the greens, cucumber, tomato, tuna, and beans in a medium bowl and toss gently to combine. In a small bowl or measuring cup, whisk together the oil, lemon juice, and vinegar. Pour the dressing over the salad and toss gently to combine. Top the salad with the avocado and season with salt and pepper to taste.

2 cups mixed greens

½ small cucumber, chopped

1 Roma tomato, chopped

½ cup low-mercury canned tuna (about 3 ounces)

¼ cup cooked cannellini beans, no salt added, or 1 organic large hard-boiled egg

½ tablespoon extra-virgin olive oil

1 tablespoon freshly squeezed lemon juice

1 tablespoon balsamic vinegar

¼ avocado, sliced

Himalayan or sea salt and freshly ground black pepper

Power Up!

ADD TO YOUR BOWL:

1 teaspoon horseradish

MEAL MATH per serving						
calories	fat	sodium	carbs	fiber	sugar	protein
350	16	90mg	25g	9g	9g	29g

KALE SALAD
WITH CITRUS SALMON

MAKES 4 SERVINGS

GF *Gluten-free*

4 (5-ounce) wild salmon fillets

3 tablespoons freshly squeezed orange juice

1 teaspoon minced fresh dill

8 cups chopped kale

2 tablespoons extra-virgin olive oil

Juice of 1 lemon

10 cherry tomatoes, halved

6 radishes, thinly sliced

2 carrots, grated

Himalayan or sea salt and freshly ground black pepper

Power Up!

TOP WITH:

1 to 2 tablespoons broccoli sprouts

Preheat the oven to 400°F.

Line a baking dish with parchment paper and place the salmon in it. Pour 2 tablespoons of the orange juice on top, sprinkle with the dill, and allow to stand at room temperature for 5 to 10 minutes. Place the baking dish in the oven and roast the salmon for 12 to 15 minutes, until it is just cooked through. Cooking time will depend on the thickness of the fish, so check on it frequently.

While the salmon is cooking, place the kale in a large bowl. In a small bowl or measuring cup, whisk together the oil and lemon juice, then pour it over the kale and toss to combine. Gently massage the kale and allow mixture to sit for 5 to 7 minutes. Add the remaining 1 tablespoon orange juice, the tomatoes, radishes, and carrots and toss gently to combine. Top the salad with the salmon, season with salt and pepper to taste, and serve.

MEAL MATH per serving						
calories	fat	sodium	carbs	fiber	sugar	protein
360	17g	135mg	18g	6g	4g	35g

STIR-FRY YOUR WAY

MAKES 2 SERVINGS

VO *Vegan option* **GF** *Gluten-free*

Heat the oil in a large skillet or wok over medium-high heat. Add the onion and garlic and sauté for 3 to 5 minutes, until softened. Add the tofu and cook until browned on all sides, 3 to 4 minutes. Add the carrot and bell pepper to the mixture and sauté for another 2 minutes. Stir in the bok choy, cook for 2 to 3 minutes, and remove the pan from the heat.

In a small saucepan, combine the water, vinegar, and tamari. Bring to a simmer and cook for 2 minutes, then stir in the tapioca mixture and cook 2 to 3 minutes more, until the sauce thickens. Pour the sauce over the veggies and tofu and serve.

1 tablespoon avocado, almond, or walnut oil

½ medium onion, sliced

2 cloves garlic, minced

12 ounces firm organic sprouted tofu, drained and patted dry, or 8 ounces organic chicken breast or grass-fed beef, cut into bite-size pieces

1 carrot, thinly sliced

1 red, yellow, or green bell pepper, cored, seeded, and chopped

4 cups chopped baby bok choy

¼ cup filtered water

2 tablespoons rice wine vinegar

1 tablespoon low-sodium tamari

1 teaspoon tapioca starch or arrowroot powder mixed with 1 tablespoon cold water

Power Up!

TOP YOUR BOWL WITH:

½-inch piece fresh ginger, peeled and minced

MEAL MATH per serving							
calories	*fat*	*sodium*	*carbs*	*fiber*	*sugar*	*protein*
310	17g	430mg	18g	5g	7g	23g

CHICKPEA SALAD

MAKES 2 SERVINGS

V *Vegan*   GF *Gluten-free*

1½ cups cooked chickpeas, no salt added

3 cups arugula or other dark, leafy greens

1 cup halved cherry tomatoes

1 medium cucumber, chopped

⅓ cup chopped fresh parsley

2 tablespoons chopped fresh mint

Juice of 1 lemon

1 tablespoon extra-virgin olive oil

Pinch of Himalayan or sea salt and freshly ground black pepper

Power Up!

TOP YOUR BOWL WITH:

1 tablespoon hemp seeds

Combine the chickpeas, arugula, tomatoes, cucumber, parsley, and mint in a large bowl. In a small bowl, whisk together the lemon juice, oil, and salt and pepper. Pour the dressing over the salad and toss gently to combine.

MEAL MATH per serving						
calories	fat	sodium	carbs	fiber	sugar	protein
310	9g	65mg	45g	10g	7g	13g

TOFU SCRAMBLE

MAKES 2 SERVINGS

V Vegan GF Gluten-free

Heat the oil in a large pan over medium heat. Add the onion and garlic and sauté for 3 to 5 minutes, until softened. Add the bell pepper, tomatoes, and mushrooms and sauté another 3 minutes. Add the kale, cover the pan, and steam for 2 minutes. Move the veggies to one side of the pan, add the tofu to the other side, and sauté for 2 minutes. Add the cumin, chili powder, and turmeric and stir to combine. Season with salt and pepper to taste and serve.

1 tablespoon extra-virgin olive oil

¼ medium red onion, thinly sliced

1 clove garlic, minced

1 red bell pepper, cored, seeded, and thinly sliced

2 Roma tomatoes, chopped

1 cup sliced mushrooms

2 cups chopped kale

12 ounces firm organic sprouted tofu, drained and patted dry, and cut into bite-size pieces

½ teaspoon ground cumin

¼ teaspoon chili powder

¼ teaspoon ground turmeric

Himalayan or sea salt and freshly ground black pepper

Power Up!

ADD TO THE PAN:

¼ teaspoon red pepper flakes (along with other spices)

MEAL MATH per serving						
calories	fat	sodium	carbs	fiber	sugar	protein
290	18g	55mg	18g	4g	5g	21g

FISH IN A PACKET

MAKES 1 SERVING

GF *Gluten-free*

2 cups mixed vegetables of your choice, such as zucchini or yellow squash, broccoli, asparagus, mushrooms, and cherry tomatoes, chopped

1 (5-ounce) fish fillet of your choice, such as black cod or wild salmon

1 tablespoon extra-virgin olive oil

Himalayan or sea salt and freshly ground black pepper

1 lemon, sliced into ¼-inch-thick rounds

Power Up!

ADD TO FISH, ALONG WITH LEMON SLICES:

⅛ cup parsley or herb of your choice, chopped

Preheat the oven to 375°F.

Line a baking sheet with parchment paper. Spread out the veggies on one end of the baking sheet and the fish fillet on the other. Brush both the salmon and the veg lightly with oil and season with salt and pepper. Top the salmon with the lemon slices. Fold the parchment over the salmon and veggies and, beginning at one end, crimp the edges to seal it completely, so you'll wind up with a semicircle-shaped packet.

Bake for 12 to 15 minutes, until cooked through. Cooking time will depend on the thickness of the salmon, so check on it frequently. Carefully open the packet to release the steam and serve.

MEAL MATH per serving						
calories	*fat*	*sodium*	*carbs*	*fiber*	*sugar*	*protein*
430	29g	100mg	21g	8g	3g	32g

Mix-and-Match Meals

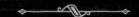

Here are some DIY plates for when you want more versatility. Tip: You can double the protein recipes and use the leftover serving to top soups that call for added protein. (And you know you're always welcome to throw in more vegetables!)

The method couldn't be simpler: Just select one of the vegetable options, pair it with a protein, include your healthful fat of choice—and be sure to power it up with spices and powerfoods. Easy, right?

If you're in a salad mood, go ahead and use 2 cups of the greens of your choice (no iceberg allowed!) plus another low-starch veg.

STEWED GREEN BEANS WITH TOMATOES

MAKES 4 SERVINGS

V Vegan GF Gluten-free

2 teaspoons extra-virgin olive oil

1 small onion, chopped

3 cloves garlic, minced

1 pound green beans, ends removed

4 Roma tomatoes, chopped

1 teaspoon minced fresh oregano or ½ teaspoon dried

1 teaspoon minced fresh thyme or ½ teaspoon dried

4 large basil leaves, thinly sliced

Himalayan or sea salt and freshly ground black pepper

Heat the oil in a large skillet over medium-high heat. Add the onion and garlic and sauté for 3 to 5 minutes, until softened. Add the green beans, tomatoes, and herbs and simmer on medium-low heat, partially covered, for 10 to 12 minutes, or until the beans are tender. Lightly season with salt and pepper.

Power Up!

ADD TO THE SKILLET:

½ teaspoon turmeric (along with the herbs)

MEAL MATH per serving						
calories	fat	sodium	carbs	fiber	sugar	protein
70	1g	15mg	15g	5g	7g	3g

SIMPLE SAUTÉED SPINACH

MAKES 2 SERVINGS

V *Vegan* **GF** *Gluten-free*

Heat the oil in a large skillet over medium-high heat. Add the garlic and sauté for 3 to 5 minutes, until softened. Add the spinach and water and sauté 3 to 4 minutes more, until the spinach has wilted. Carefully drain the excess liquid from the spinach and continue sautéing for 3 to 4 minutes. Season with salt and pepper to taste.

1 teaspoon extra-virgin olive oil

2 cloves garlic, minced

8 cups baby spinach

¼ cup filtered water

Himalayan or sea salt and freshly ground black pepper

Power Up!

ADD TO YOUR BOWL:

1 tablespoon freshly grated lemon zest

MEAL MATH per serving						
calories	fat	sodium	carbs	fiber	sugar	protein
50	3g	95mg	5g	3g	<1g	4g

SPICY MANDARIN MARINATED ZUCCHINI

MAKES 4 SERVINGS

V Vegan GF Gluten-free

1 teaspoon low-sodium tamari

Zest and juice of 1 small orange

½ teaspoon ground ginger

¼ teaspoon ground cayenne pepper

1 clove garlic, minced

¼ teaspoon ground turmeric (optional)

4 medium zucchini, sliced

1½ teaspoons extra-virgin olive oil

Himalayan or sea salt and freshly ground black pepper

Place the tamari, orange zest and juice, ginger, cayenne, garlic, and, if using, the turmeric in a large bowl and whisk together. Add the zucchini and toss to coat. Cover the bowl and allow the mixture to marinate for about 15 minutes. Heat the oil in a large skillet over medium-high heat. Add the marinated zucchini, including any excess marinade, and sauté for 6 to 8 minutes, until the zucchini is tender but not mushy. Season with salt and pepper to taste.

Power Up!

ADD TO THE
MIXING BOWL:

1 tablespoon nutritional yeast (along with the spices)

MEAL MATH per serving						
calories	fat	sodium	carbs	fiber	sugar	protein
70	2.5g	55mg	10g	3g	7g	3g

BALSAMIC-ROASTED TOMATOES

MAKES 4 SERVINGS

V *Vegan* **GF** *Gluten-free*

Preheat the broiler.

In a small bowl, whisk together the oil and vinegar. Place the tomatoes on a baking sheet, add the vinegar and oil mixture, and toss to coat. Broil for 15 to 20 minutes, until the tomatoes burst and darken slightly. Season with salt and pepper to taste.

1½ teaspoons extra-virgin olive oil

3 tablespoons balsamic vinegar

4 cups grape tomatoes

Himalayan or sea salt and freshly ground black pepper

Power Up!

ADD TO THE TOMATOES:

1 tablespoon chopped fresh basil (sprinkled on top prior to roasting)

MEAL MATH per serving						
calories	fat	sodium	carbs	fiber	sugar	protein
70	4g	15mg	8g	2g	4g	2g

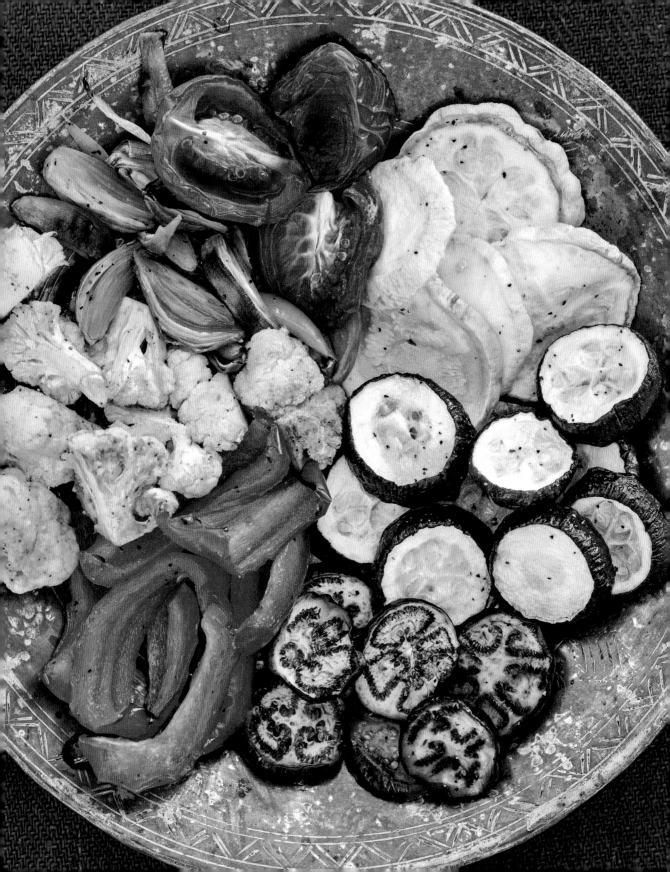

SIMPLE ROASTED VEG

MAKES 4 TO 6 SERVINGS

V *Vegan*   **GF** *Gluten-free*

Preheat the oven to 400° F.

Toss the veg in a bowl with the oil and the salt and pepper to taste. Line a baking sheet with parchment paper and spread out the veg and garlic cloves and onion, if using. Roasting times for your veg are listed here:

10–15 minutes
Asparagus, tough ends removed
Broccoli, cut into florets
Cauliflower, cut into florets
Yellow squash, sliced
Zucchini, sliced

15–20 minutes
Cherry tomatoes
Mushrooms, cut in half lengthwise

20–30 minutes
Baby artichokes, trimmed and cut in half
Brussels sprouts, trimmed and cut in half
Carrots, sliced
Eggplant, sliced

6 cups of vegetables
(choose any from the list)

2 tablespoons olive oil, walnut oil, or avocado oil

Himalayan or sea salt and freshly ground black pepper

4 garlic cloves (optional)

1 medium onion, sliced
(optional)

Power Up!

ADD TO THE VEG:

1 teaspoon turmeric or
1 teaspoon cumin (along with the salt and pepper)

MEAL MATH per serving						
calories	*fat*	*sodium*	*carbs*	*fiber*	*sugar*	*protein*
70	6g	20mg	5g	2g	3g	2g

CAULIFLOWER FRIED "RICE"

MAKES 4 SERVINGS

V Vegan **GF** Gluten-free

2 teaspoons coconut oil

1 small onion, chopped

2 cloves garlic, minced

1 red bell pepper, cored, seeded, and chopped

1 yellow bell pepper, cored, seeded, and chopped

1 orange bell pepper, cored, seeded, and chopped

Head of cauliflower, grated in a food processor until it resembles rice

½ teaspoon ground cumin

½ teaspoon ground turmeric

Himalayan or sea salt and freshly ground black pepper

Heat the oil in a large pan over medium-high heat. Add the onion, garlic, and peppers and sauté 3 to 5 minutes, until softened. Add the cauliflower, cumin, and turmeric. Cover the pan and cook until the veg are slightly softened but still crunchy, about 5 minutes. Season with salt and pepper.

Power Up!

TOP YOUR BOWL WITH:

1 to 2 tablespoons kimchi

MEAL MATH per serving						
calories	fat	sodium	carbs	fiber	sugar	protein
90	3g	50mg	15g	5g	7g	4g

Step 2: Add a Protein

POACHED CHICKEN WITH LEMON

MAKES 4 SERVINGS

GF *Gluten-free*

Place the broth, lemon slices, rosemary, and pepper in a large pot or deep pan over high heat and bring to a boil. Add the chicken breasts and reduce the heat to very low and simmer gently for 12 to 15 minutes, or until cooked through. The chicken breasts will spring back lightly when poked. Do not overcook!

4 cups low-sodium vegetable broth

1 lemon, sliced

2 sprigs fresh rosemary

Pinch of freshly ground black pepper

4 (5-ounce) boneless, skinless organic chicken breasts

Power Up!

ADD TO THE POT:

½ teaspoon cayenne pepper (with the broth mixture)

MEAL MATH per serving						
calories	fat	sodium	carbs	fiber	sugar	protein
160	3.5g	160mg	0g	0g	0g	30g

SPEEDY BROILED SALMON

MAKES 1 SERVING

GF *Gluten-free*

1 (5-ounce) wild salmon fillet

½ teaspoon extra-virgin olive oil

¼ teaspoon dried Italian herbs or whatever dried herbs you have on hand

Pinch of Himalayan or sea salt

Pinch of freshly ground black pepper

Power Up!

ADD TO THE SALMON
BEFORE SERVING:

1 tablespoon freshly squeezed lemon juice

Preheat the broiler.

Line a baking sheet with parchment paper and place the salmon on it skin side down. In a small bowl or measuring cup, whisk together the oil, Italian herbs, and salt and pepper and brush the mixture over the top of the salmon. Broil for 5 to 7 minutes, until cooked through. Cooking time will depend on the thickness of the fish, so check on it frequently.

Remove the salmon from the oven and serve.

MEAL MATH per serving						
calories	fat	sodium	carbs	fiber	sugar	protein
230	11g	65mg	0g	0g	0g	28g

GARLIC AND LEMON SAUTÉED JUMBO SHRIMP

MAKES 1 SERVING

GF *Gluten-free*

Toss the shrimp, paprika, and 1 tablespoon of the lemon juice together in a bowl. Heat the oil in a small skillet over medium-high heat. Add the shrimp and garlic and sauté for 4 to 5 minutes, or until the shrimp turns opaque. Add the lemon zest and remaining juice and sauté 1 minute more, until shrimp is just pink and cooked through. Season with salt and pepper to taste.

5 ounces fresh or frozen shrimp, peeled and deveined

¼ teaspoon smoked paprika

Zest and juice of 1 small lemon

1 teaspoon extra-virgin olive oil

1 clove garlic, minced

Himalayan or sea salt and freshly ground black pepper

Power Up!

ADD TO THE SKILLET:

1 tablespoon minced fresh parsley (along with the garlic)

MEAL MATH per serving						
calories	*fat*	*sodium*	*carbs*	*fiber*	*sugar*	*protein*
170	2.5g	340mg	6g	0g	1g	28g

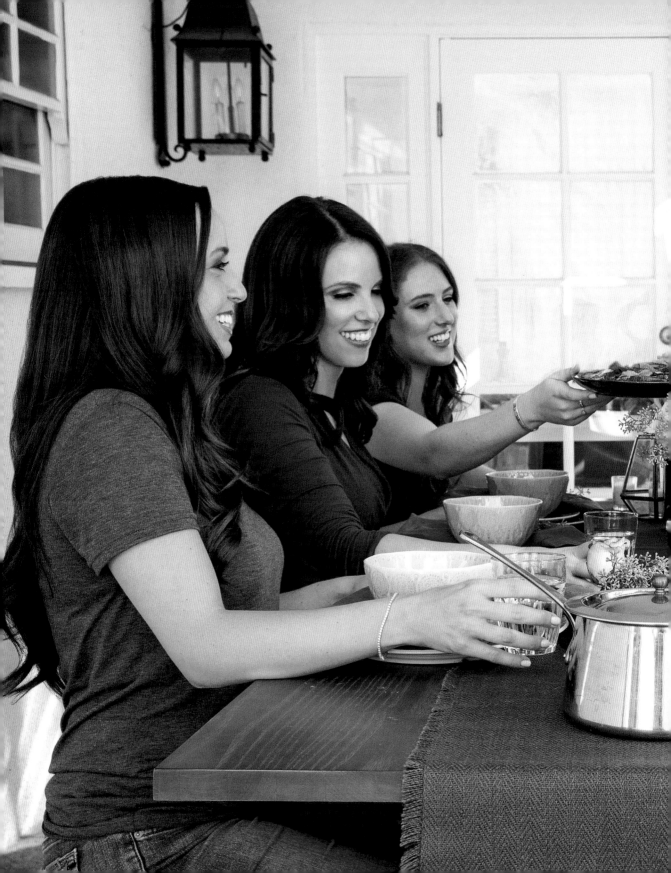

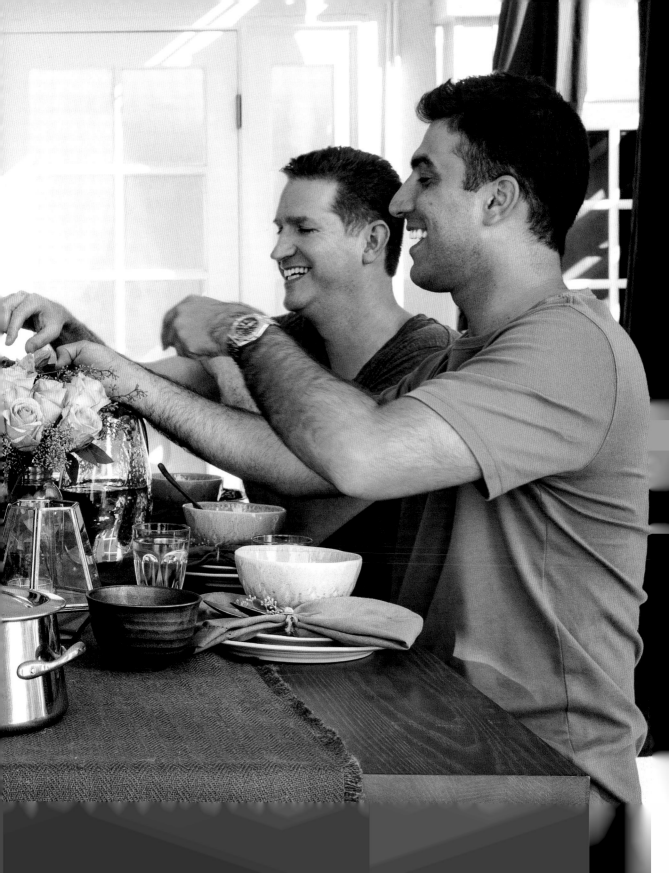

ZESTY EDAMAME–JUST ADD GREENS!

MAKES 3 SERVINGS

V *Vegan* **GF** *Gluten-free*

3 cups frozen organic edamame, thawed

1 tablespoon low-sodium tamari

2 cloves garlic, minced

½-inch piece fresh ginger, peeled and minced

1 green onion (white and light green parts only), thinly sliced

Zest and juice of 1 orange

1 tablespoon avocado oil

½ teaspoon sesame oil

Pinch of freshly ground black pepper

Place the edamame, tamari, garlic, ginger, green onion, orange zest and juice, avocado and sesame oils, and pepper in a bowl and toss together. Cover and refrigerate for 15 minutes before eating.

Power Up!

ADD TO THE BOWL:

1 teaspoon toasted sesame seeds

Sprinkle of dried nori flakes

MEAL MATH per serving						
calories	fat	sodium	carbs	fiber	sugar	protein
190	11g	160mg	14g	6g	5g	13g

SPICED CHICKPEAS

MAKES 4 SERVINGS

V *Vegan* **GF** *Gluten-free*

Heat a large saucepan over high heat. Add the oil, turmeric, cumin, paprika, black pepper, and cayenne. Season with salt, if using. Add the chickpeas and cook for 7 to 10 minutes, stirring frequently, or until slightly crisp. Serve warm or cold.

1 tablespoon coconut oil

1½ teaspoons ground turmeric

1 teaspoon ground cumin

1 teaspoon paprika

¼ teaspoon freshly ground black pepper

Pinch of ground cayenne pepper

Himalayan or sea salt (optional)

3 cups cooked chickpeas, no salt added

Power Up!

ADD TO THE SAUCEPAN:

2 tablespoons nutritional yeast (along with the other spices)

MEAL MATH per serving						
calories	fat	sodium	carbs	fiber	sugar	protein
230	5g	45mg	36g	8g	2g	11g

EGG WHITE-ISH SALAD

MAKES 4 SERVINGS

V *Vegan*   **GF** *Gluten-free*

12 hard-boiled organic eggs, all whites and 3 yolks reserved

4 tablespoons Basic Hummus (page 207) or ½ avocado

½ teaspoon Dijon mustard

¼ cup red onion, chopped

⅛ teaspoon turmeric

Himalayan or sea salt and freshly ground black pepper

Power Up!

ADD TO THE BOWL:

1 teaspoon paprika (along with the other spices)

Chop the egg whites and yolks and place in a small bowl. Stir in the hummus, mustard, onion, turmeric, and salt and pepper.

MEAL MATH	*per serving*					
calories	*fat*	*sodium*	*carbs*	*fiber*	*sugar*	*protein*
150	8g	220mg	4g	2g	2g	16g

Step 3: Add 1 serving of Fat

Because your mix-and-match veg and protein choices most likely already include some fat, you may not need this second serving.

SESAME KALE PESTO

MAKES 20 SERVINGS (SERVING SIZE: 1 TABLESPOON)

V Vegan   **GF** Gluten-free

Place the kale, garlic, sesame seeds, and oil in a high-powered blender and puree until smooth. Season with salt and pepper to taste.

4 cups chopped kale

1 clove garlic

2 tablespoons sesame seeds

2 tablespoons extra-virgin olive oil

Himalayan or sea salt and freshly ground black pepper

MEAL MATH per serving						
calories	fat	sodium	carbs	fiber	sugar	protein
25	2g	5mg	2g	0g	0g	1g

POWERFOOD PESTO

MAKES 20 SERVINGS (SERVING SIZE: 1 TABLESPOON)

V Vegan **GF** Gluten-free

1 cup fresh basil leaves

1 cup fresh parsley leaves

2 cups baby spinach

3 cups roughly chopped broccoli

¼ cup sunflower seeds

1 clove garlic, rough chopped

4 tablespoons extra-virgin olive oil

Himalayan or sea salt and freshly ground black pepper

Place the basil, parsley, spinach, broccoli, sunflower seeds, garlic, and oil in a high-powered blender and puree until smooth. Season with salt and pepper to taste.

MEAL MATH	per serving					
calories	fat	sodium	carbs	fiber	sugar	protein
40	3.5g	10mg	2g	1g	0g	1g

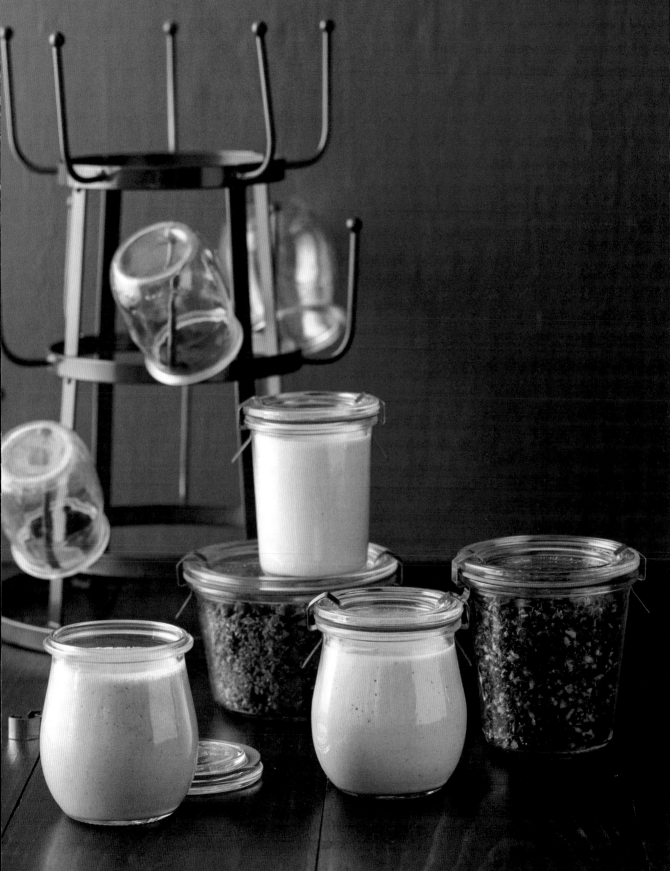

CASHEW CRÈME

MAKES 8 SERVINGS (SERVING SIZE: 1 TABLESPOON)

V *Vegan* **GF** *Gluten-free*

½ cup raw cashews

½ cup filtered water

1 teaspoon freshly squeezed lemon juice

1 clove garlic

1 tablespoon nutritional yeast (optional)

Place the cashews, filtered water, lemon juice, garlic, and nutritional yeast, if using, in a high-powered blender and puree for 45 to 60 seconds, until creamy.

Note: You can also soak the cashews in hot water for 30 minutes, drain, and then blend for a smoother consistency.

2 tablespoons chopped fresh basil

1 tablespoons chopped fresh parsley

½ cup baby spinach

GREEN CRÈME

Add basil, parsley, and spinach to the basic Cashew Crème before processing.

1 small red chile pepper, such as cayenne or jalapeño, seeded and finely diced

½ roasted fresh or jarred red bell pepper

RED CRÈME

Add chile and bell pepper to the basic Cashew Crème before processing.

1 heaping tablespoon Ceylon cinnamon

1 teaspoon raw honey (optional)

CINNAMON SWEET CRÈME

Omit the lemon juice, garlic, and nutritional yeast from the basic Cashew Crème and add the cinnamon and the honey, if using, before processing.

MEAL MATH per serving						
calories	*fat*	*sodium*	*carbs*	*fiber*	*sugar*	*protein*
60	4.5g	0mg	4g	0g	<1g	2g

BASIC HUMMUS

MAKES 6 SERVINGS (SERVING SIZE: ¼ CUP)

V Vegan   **GF** Gluten-free

Combine the chickpeas, garlic, oil, lemon juice, tahini, and cumin in a food processor or high-powered blender until fully incorporated. Add the filtered water 1 tablespoon at a time as needed to reach desired consistency; you may not need to use it all. Season with salt and pepper to taste.

1½ cups cooked chickpeas, no salt added

1 clove garlic

¼ cup extra-virgin olive oil

2 tablespoons freshly squeezed lemon juice

2 tablespoons tahini

1 teaspoon cumin

¼ cup filtered water

Himalayan or sea salt and freshly ground black pepper

MEAL MATH per serving						
calories	fat	sodium	carbs	fiber	sugar	protein
170	13g	170mg	10g	3g	0g	4g

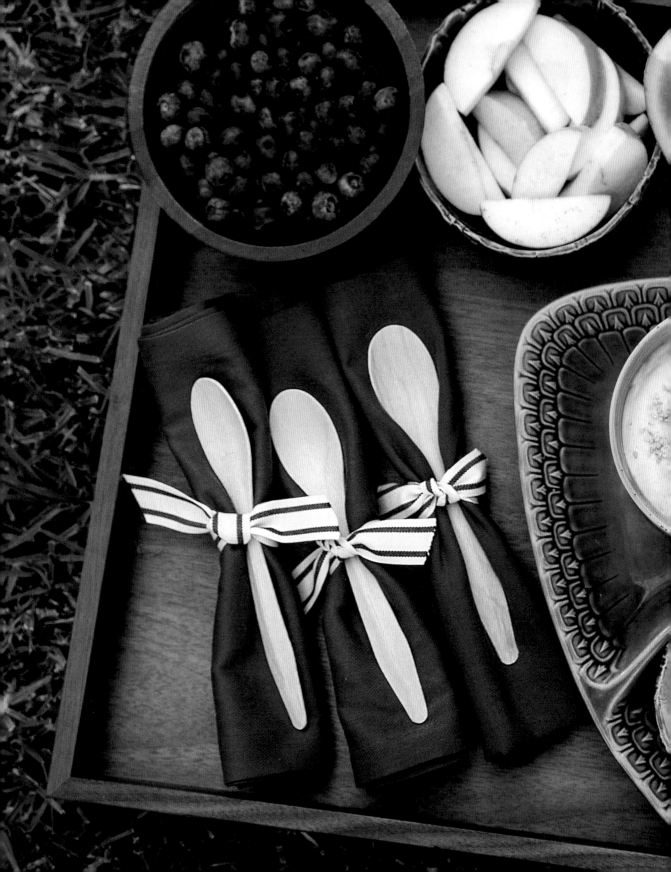

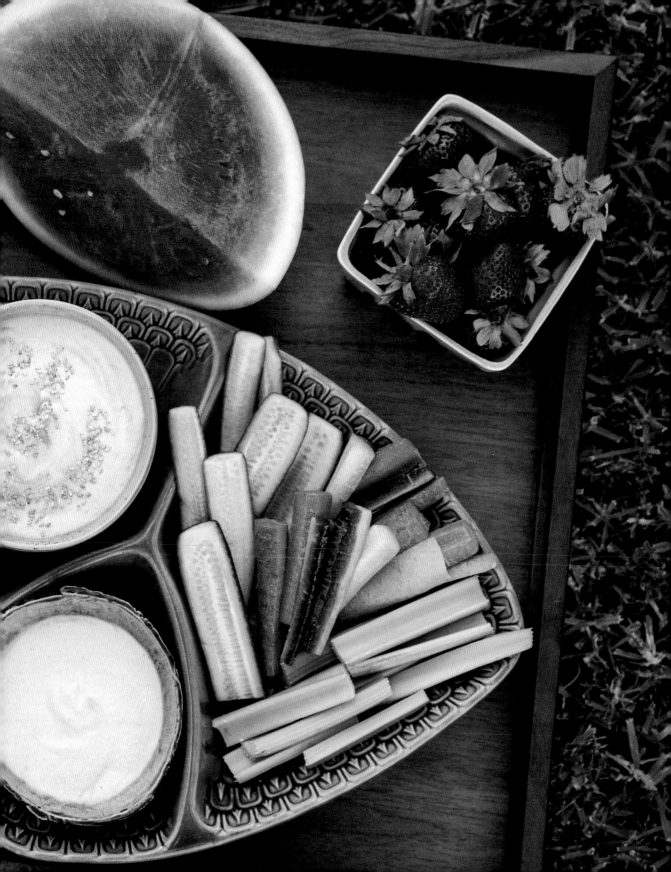

CLASSIC VINAIGRETTE

MAKES 18 SERVINGS (SERVING SIZE: 1 TABLESPOON)

V *Vegan* **GF** *Gluten-free*

6 tablespoons extra-virgin olive oil

3 tablespoons balsamic vinegar

3 tablespoons chopped shallots

2 tablespoons Dijon mustard

4 tablespoons freshly squeezed lemon juice

¼ teaspoon freshly ground black pepper

½ teaspoon Himalayan or sea salt (optional)

Combine the oil, vinegar, shallots, mustard, lemon juice, pepper, and salt, if using, in a blender until fully incorporated.

MEAL MATH per serving						
calories	fat	sodium	carbs	fiber	sugar	protein
45	5g	85mg	1g	0g	0g	0g

CARROT SESAME DRESSING

MAKES 24 SERVINGS (SERVING SIZE: 1 TABLESPOON)

GF *Gluten-free*

2 cups chopped carrots

½ cup freshly squeezed orange juice (1 to 2 oranges)

4 tablespoons freshly squeezed lime juice

4 tablespoons avocado oil

1 teaspoon sesame oil

1-inch piece ginger, peeled and minced

1 tablespoon raw honey (optional)

Combine the carrots, orange juice, lime juice, avocado and sesame oils, ginger, and raw honey, if using, in a blender. Puree until almost smooth.

MEAL MATH per serving						
calories	fat	sodium	carbs	fiber	sugar	protein
30	2.5g	5mg	2g	0g	0g	0g

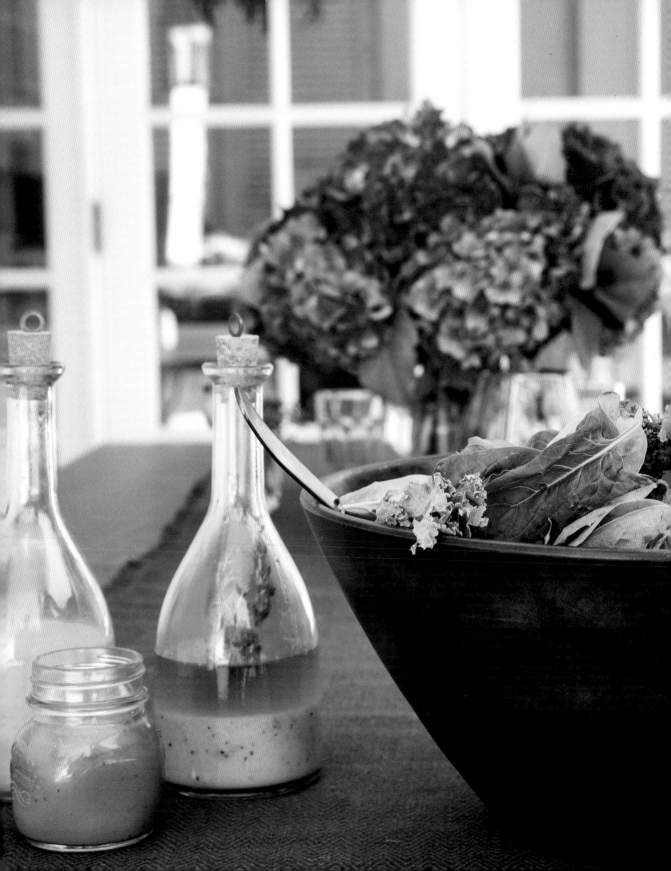

LEMON DRESSING

MAKES 24 SERVINGS (SERVING SIZE: 1 TABLESPOON)

GF *Gluten-free*

¾ cup freshly squeezed lemon juice (4 to 5 lemons)

10 tablespoons extra-virgin olive oil

4 teaspoons Dijon mustard

1 tablespoon raw honey

1 sprig fresh oregano

¼ teaspoon freshly ground black pepper

¼ teaspoon Himalayan or sea salt (optional)

Combine the lemon juice, oil, mustard, raw honey, oregano, pepper, and salt, if using, in a mason jar. Shake vigorously before using.

MEAL MATH per serving						
calories	fat	sodium	carbs	fiber	sugar	protein
60	6g	35mg	1g	0g	0g	0g

Step 4: Power Up!

Add more power to your meals with my spice and powerfood toppers on pages 92–96.

Enjoy!

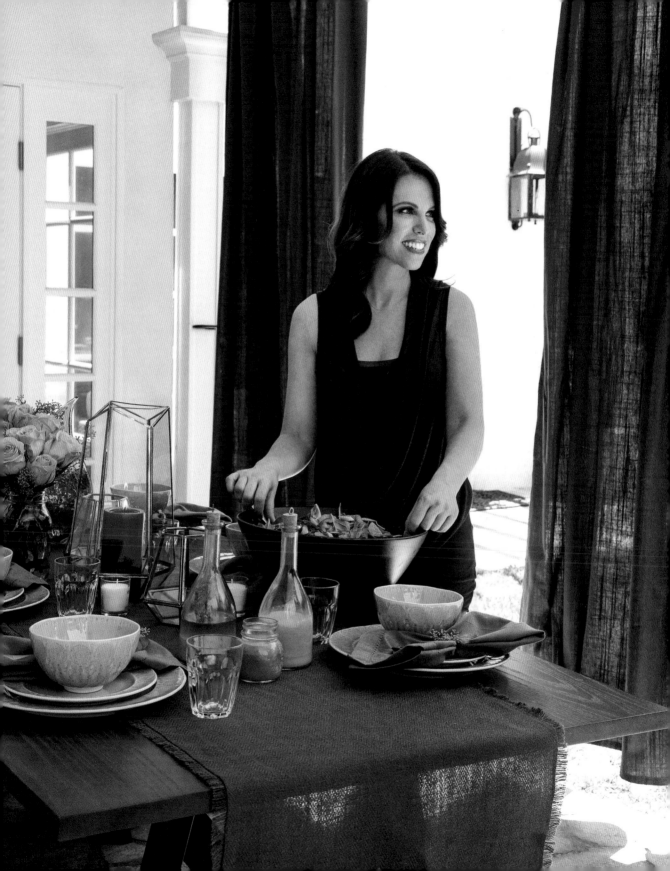

Dessert Plates

GREEK YOGURT FROZEN POPS

MAKES 6 ICE POPS (SERVING SIZE: 1 ICE POP)

VO *Vegan option* **GF** *Gluten-free*

In a medium bowl, combine the yogurt, milk, chia seeds, and vanilla. Gently add in your choice of berries. Scoop the mixture into ice pop molds and place in the freezer to set, approximately 3 hours.

1 cup organic plain 2% Greek yogurt or Vegan Yogurt (page 135)

½ cup unsweetened plant-based milk (see page 139)

1 tablespoon chia seeds

½ teaspoon pure vanilla extract

½ cup chopped berries, such as blueberries, strawberries, and/ or raspberries

MEAL MATH per serving						
calories	fat	sodium	carbs	fiber	sugar	protein
50	1.5g	35mg	3g	2g	2g	4g

RAW CACAO BLISS BALLS

MAKES 12 BALLS (SERVING SIZE: 1 BALL)

V *Vegan* **GF** *Gluten-free*

1 cup dates, pitted

¾ cup raw almonds or nuts of your choice

¼ cup coconut oil

⅓ cup raw cacao powder

1 tablespoon chia seeds

½ cup unsweetened coconut flakes

⅛ teaspoon Himalayan or sea salt

Filtered water for rolling (optional)

Soften dates by soaking them in warm water for 10 to 15 minutes. Place the almonds, coconut oil, cacao powder, chia seeds, coconut flakes, and salt in a food processor and blend. Drain the dates and add them in; blend until fully combined. If the mixture is dry, try adding a tablespoon of filtered water. Roll the paste into 12 balls and refrigerate in an airtight container until semi-firm. Keeps for about 1 week in the refrigerator.

MEAL MATH per serving						
calories	fat	sodium	carbs	fiber	sugar	protein
150	11g	55mg	11g	4g	7g	3g

RAW COOKIE DOUGH BALLS

MAKES 12 BALLS (SERVING SIZE: 1 BALL)

V Vegan **GF** Gluten-free

Place the cashews, oats, cinnamon, and salt in a food processor and pulse until you reach a fine, meal-like consistency (but not cashew butter). Add the vanilla and maple syrup and process until you reach a dough consistency. Place the dough in a bowl and fold in the cacao nibs. Roll into 12 balls and refrigerate in an airtight container until semi-firm. Keeps for about 1 week in the refrigerator.

1 cup raw cashews

½ cup gluten-free rolled oats

½ teaspoon Ceylon cinnamon

¼ teaspoon Himalayan or sea salt

1 teaspoon pure vanilla extract

3 tablespoons pure maple syrup

¼ cup raw cacao nibs

MEAL MATH per serving						
calories	fat	sodium	carbs	fiber	sugar	protein
110	7g	50mg	8g	2g	4g	3g

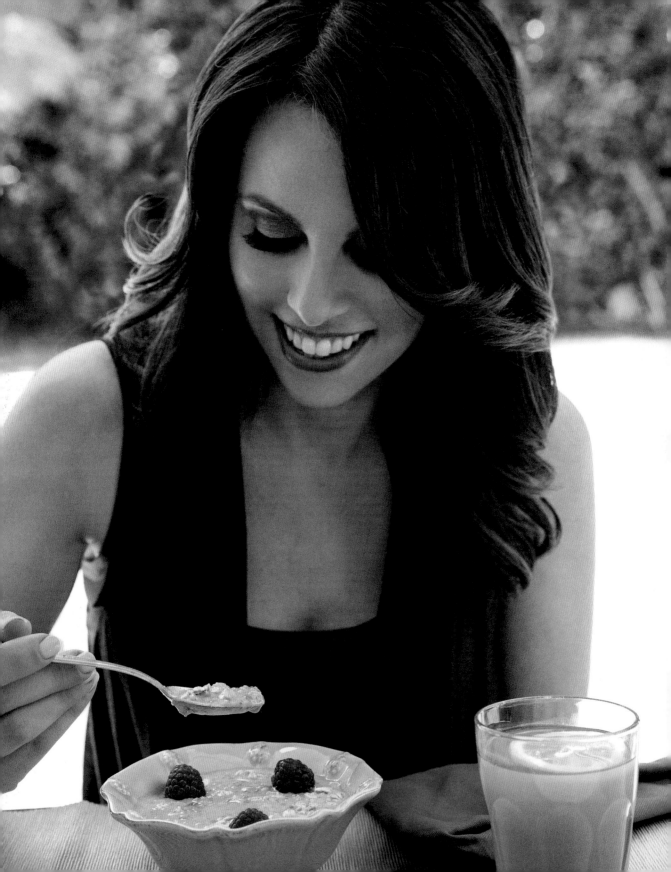

4.
Maintain Me for Life

A LIFESTYLE YOU CAN STICK TO FOREVER

Welcome to the new *you*. Congrats on finishing the 24-Day Transformation!

You've shed pounds, changed the way you think about what you put into your body, and I bet you're *feeling* the difference. I'm going to help you hold on to that feeling—for life.

Being able to maintain the investment you've made in yourself is the true definition of weight-loss success—and in this chapter you'll learn how to continue incorporating souping into your everyday lifestyle in an effective, sustainable way. In other words: You won't need to do anything drastically new or complex. You already have a solid foundation with my Rule of 3, but now I'm expanding the clean food calories and ingredients list to give you even more options to choose from.

Maintain Me for Life Principles

- 85 percent of the time, stick to the Rule of 3.

- 15 percent of the time, you can step out of bounds a little—like if you're having a special dinner out.

- Don't let go of the clean-eating principle. Continue eating only foods with easily ID-able ingredients that yield a return on your health.

- Keep souping several times a week. It's a habit I don't want you to break—and it's such a simple way to pack in nutrients and control caloric intake.

- Spot-check all your meals and snacks to make sure they follow the Rule of 3. That never goes away.

Now let me help you master putting meals together on your own.

Breakfast

Nothing changes from the 24-Day Transformation. I still want you to . . .

Start with the A.M. riser. Feel free to have your organic coffee afterward, but don't slip into old habits—like adding sugar or flavored creamers to your cup. Now that you've lost the weight and learned the importance of eating real, wholesome foods, keep it clean!

Then build your breakfast around the Rule of 3:

1. *Fiber Up:* Get at least 10 grams of fiber.
2. *Plant 1:* Include at least 1 serving of produce.
3. *Eye Cals:* Limit this meal to 350 "real food" calories—max.

You may add in more protein, if you like. Watch the total calories, though!

Lunch and Dinner

I'm opening up more options. Take a look.

Make sure your meal—soup or plated—still fulfills the lunch and dinner Rule of 3:

1. *Veg Out:* Load up on about 2 cups of low-starch veggies.
2. *Go Pro:* Include 1 serving of protein.
3. *Fatten Up:* Add 1 to 2 servings of fat.

Here's what else you get: Add 1 serving of a complex carb or high-starch vegetable.
Start by having it at *either* lunch or dinner—but not both—and see how it goes for a couple of weeks. If your weight doesn't creep up at all, then go ahead and have a serving at lunch *and* dinner.

Want to add some carbs into your souping experience? Check out More Soups for You! recipes on pages 225–235. Or, if you're the DIY type, simply add a serving of one of the complex carbs or starchy vegetables listed next to your soups and plated meals.

HERE'S WHAT ONE SERVING OF COMPLEX CARB LOOKS LIKE:

1 SLICE WHOLE GRAIN BREAD, 80 TO 90 CALORIES
⅓ CUP COOKED BROWN RICE, QUINOA, OR FARRO, 70 TO 75 CALORIES
½ CUP COOKED WHOLE WHEAT PASTA, 85 TO 90 CALORIES
½ CUP COOKED SOBA NOODLES (OR OTHER WHOLE GRAIN NOODLE), 60 CALORIES

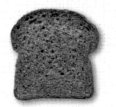

THIS IS WHAT A SERVING OF STARCHY VEGETABLE LOOKS LIKE:

1 MEDIUM POTATO, 145 CALORIES
1 MEDIUM SWEET POTATO, 103 CALORIES
1 CUP BUTTERNUT SQUASH, 82 CALORIES
½ CUP CORN, 67 CALORIES

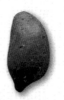

Afternoon Snack

Now that you're a pro, you've earned more snacking rights. I'm tweaking the final rule—so that you can venture into a variety of wholesome, clean foods. Check out the modified Rule 3.

The Maintain Me Afternoon Snack Rule of 3:

1. *Go Low:* Limit it to 150 to 175 calories. Less is fine, but don't go above.

2. *Be Real:* Keep it clean. Stick to high-quality ingredients you can recognize.

3. *Opt In:* You can now include different types of clean foods, such as complex carbs. My favorite P.M. fill-me-up is a small baked sweet potato and a few almonds.

After Dinner

Sometimes you just want a glass of wine after a long day. Now you can go ahead and enjoy it—just don't go overboard. I recommend having one serving of alcohol—that's 5 ounces of wine (123 calories) or 1.5 ounces of distilled spirits (about 100 calories)—no more than two or three times a week.

Remember the Dessert Rule of 3 Guidelines:

1. *Check In:* Ask yourself if you really need it.

2. *Go Low:* Keep it under 150 calories.

3. *Be Real:* Keep it clean.

Now enjoy a drink or a natural treat—but not both.

A Few More Things to Know Before You Go

1. It's okay to take an occasional food vacation. I always prescribe food vacays to my clients—they're necessary! Whether you're dining out or just having a nice meal at home, it's fine to be a *little* more liberal once in a while—meaning, go ahead and sample a natural yet decadent dessert or an interesting appetizer (think a shared tuna tartare on crispy rice crackers, not fried mozzarella sticks). Enjoy it! But don't abuse it. Just like any vacay, come back to your day-to-day feeling ready to jump right back in.

2. Spot-check, spot-check, spot-check. Although you get to be a bit more adventurous, never forget the rules from this plan. If you ever feel lost or sidetracked, you can always go back to the 24-Day Transformation.

Quick Questions

What if I notice processed food slipping back in?

Get your mind back into pure detox mode—and redo *just* the 3-Day Restart. What I find with my clients is that the total commitment phase is the strongest push on the swing I can give to get them back into full clean-eating mode. Feeling the empowerment of completing the 3-Day Restart is great motivation to regain momentum toward a clean eating lifestyle.

If I start gaining weight, what do I do?

Take an honest look at what might be tripping you up, which is usually the stuff you love and find hardest to limit—or the random bites you steal throughout the day. Try keeping track of what you're eating for a week via old-fashioned pen and paper or an app. If the culprit is an overabundance of carbs, try cutting back on either one or both optional servings at lunch and dinner. And make sure portion sizes haven't crept up. If those changes don't do the trick, go back to the 24-Day Transformation. It will give you the framework you need to take the weight off and get you back on the right path.

How do I spot-check when eating lunch or dinner out?

Ask yourself if what you're about to order fulfills the Rule of 3:

- *Will you be getting about 2 cups of veg?*
- *Do you have enough—or too much—protein?* One 4-ounce serving of protein is around the size of a computer mouse.
- *What's the fat situation like?* Remember: Fat is used to cook foods that are sautéed and seared, plus it's in the nuts, sauces, and dressings that top your dish. Many times both your fat servings are more than accounted for thanks to a heavy-handed chef!

Be sure to ask for the nuts, sauces, and dressings on the side. Then *you* own the power of controlling the fats so you don't overdose.

• **Check the carbs.** Are they complex—and how many servings are they giving you?

Don't be afraid to ask for modifications or to pack extra portions in a to-go box before you dig in. And remember the Rule of 3 for breakfasts, snacks, and desserts. Do this at every eating occasion and it'll become so natural that you won't even really think about it—you'll automatically do it as you plate or bowl your meals.

Speaking of bowls . . . turn the next page for a whole new world of soups that's now open to you.

More Soups for You!

Each recipe in this section takes a classic comfort soup and amplifies it with a clean, wholesome twist. You're more than welcome to try these recipes now that you've made it to the Maintenance phase. Take note that these soups, with the exception of Pho Real, do not meet my complete meal requirements, but feel free to enjoy them as your 175-calorie-and-under snack.

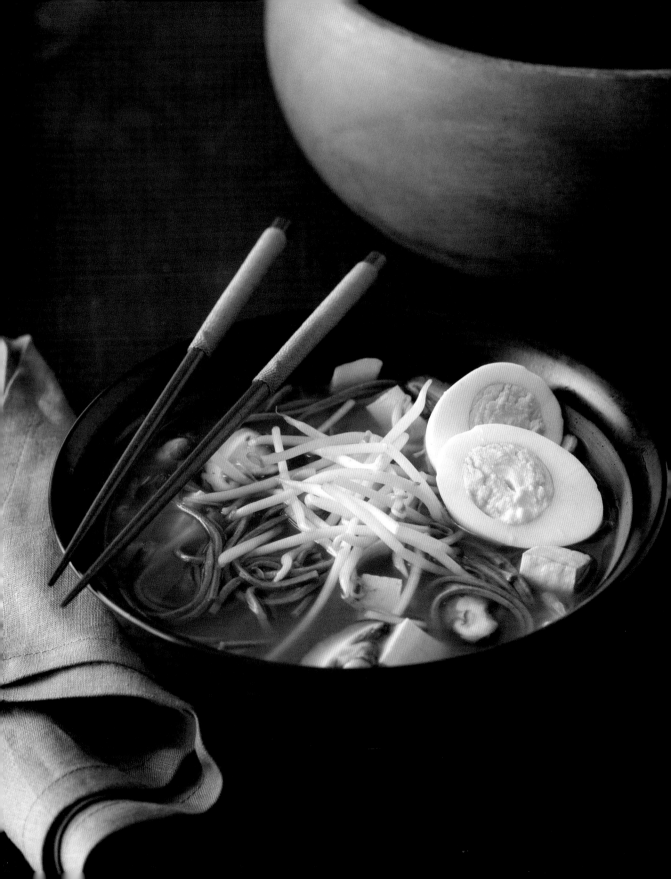

Pho Real:
CLEAN SESAME SOBA

MAKES 8 SERVINGS (SERVING SIZE: 1 CUP)

VO *Vegan option* **GF** *Gluten-free*

Remember those noodle food autopsies on pages 10 to 13? Fear not, ramen and pho lovers, I am not going to deprive you of this flavorful broth, but go with this flipped version. It's low in sodium and loaded with fresh veggies—I'm talking crunchy bean sprouts, bok choy, spinach, and mountains of fresh herbs. During Maintenance, you can add some soba noodles, but omit the noodles if you're on the Restart or Transformation phase. And you can even make it vegan if you wish—the great thing about pho is that it's so easy to customize!

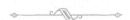

In a large pot, combine the broth, filtered water, oil, green onions, and ginger. Bring to a boil, then reduce the heat to simmer. Add in the mushrooms and simmer for 15 minutes. Stir in the bok choy, spinach, and tamari as well as any additional vegetable add-ins.

Serve the soup on top of 1 cup cooked soba noodles, add your protein of choice, and top with the garnishes.

BROTH BASE

4 cups low-sodium vegetable broth

4 cups filtered water

1 tablespoon sesame oil

3 green onions, thinly sliced

5 (1-inch) pieces fresh ginger, peeled and chopped

1 cup sliced shiitake mushrooms

2 cups chopped baby bok choy

2 cups baby spinach

2 teaspoons low-sodium tamari

4 cups cooked gluten-free soba noodles (optional)

OPTIONAL ADDITIONS

Carrots

Broccoli

Wakame (add along with mushrooms)

1 tablespoon miso paste (add along with mushrooms)

PROTEIN

4 ounces organic sprouted tofu

1 cup frozen organic edamame, thawed

1 soft-boiled organic egg

3 to 4 ounces grilled or seared wild salmon

3 to 4 ounces cooked organic chicken or grass-fed beef

GARNISHES

Bean sprouts

Jalapeño peppers, seeded and thinly sliced

Chopped fresh cilantro and basil

8 lime wedges

Chili garlic sauce or hot sauce

MEAL MATH *per serving*						
calories	fat	sodium	carbs	fiber	sugar	protein
310	12g	370mg	31g	2g	2g	23g

Gleaming:
GINGER BUTTERNUT SQUASH

MAKES 6 SERVINGS (SERVING SIZE: 1 CUP)

V *Vegan* **GF** *Gluten-free*

3 pounds butternut squash, peeled and cubed (about 8 cups)

4 large shallots, halved

2 (2-inch) pieces fresh ginger, peeled and sliced

3 tablespoons coconut oil or extra-virgin olive oil

6 cups low-sodium vegetable broth

Himalayan or sea salt and freshly ground black pepper

Not only does this creamy bowl of comfort deliver a rich velvety taste, but it supplies you with a ton of heart-healthful fiber as well as vitamins A and C for beautiful hair and skin.

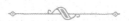

Preheat the oven to 375°F.

Place the squash, shallots, and ginger in a roasting pan. Coat with the oil, and cook for 50 minutes, or until tender, stirring occasionally. Set aside for 10 minutes to cool. Place the squash mixture in a high-powered blender along with the broth and puree until smooth. Season with salt and pepper to taste and serve.

MEAL MATH per serving						
calories	fat	sodium	carbs	fiber	sugar	protein
170	7g	150mg	27g	5g	5g	3g

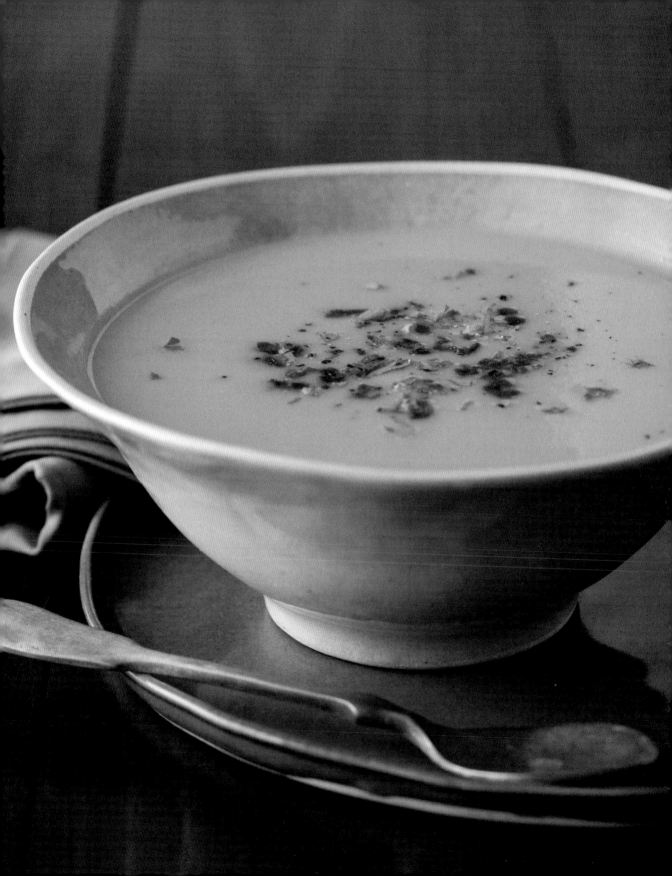

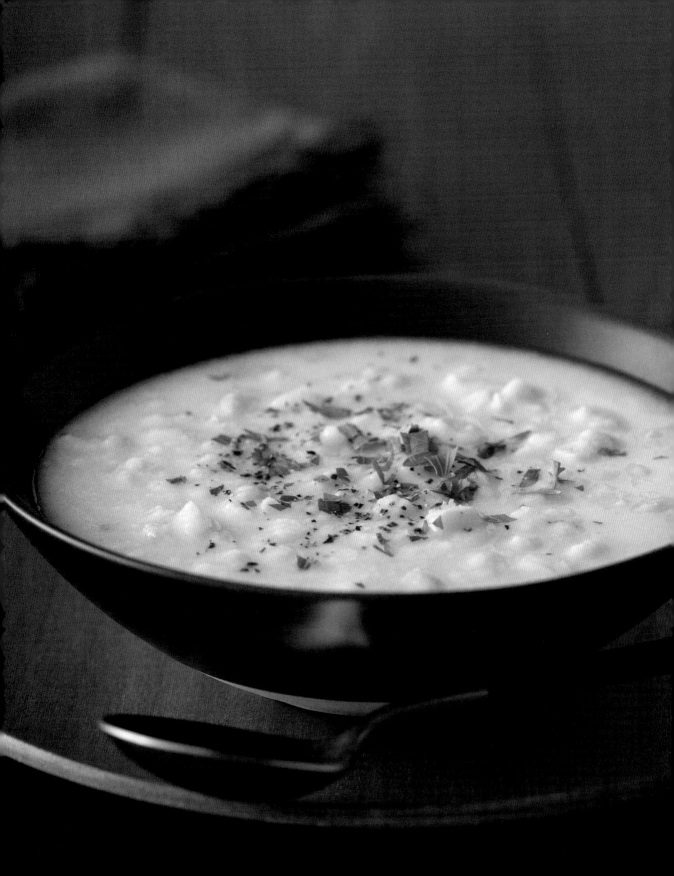

No Sweat:
CLEAN CORN CHOWDER

MAKES 8 SERVINGS (SERVING SIZE: 1 CUP)

V *Vegan* **GF** *Gluten-free*

If you thought healthful chowder was an oxymoron, I'm challenging you to think again. My take on this much-loved classic is every bit as creamy and flavorful as you're used to, but I apply a few smart swaps to keep your meal clean.

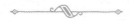

Heat ghee in a large pot over medium heat. Add the garlic and sauté for about 2 minutes. Add the onion and cook 10 minutes, until softened. Add the potatoes, corn, broth, and coconut milk and simmer for about 1 hour. Do not allow the soup to boil. Stir in the thyme and turmeric, if using, and cook 15 minutes more. Season with salt and pepper to taste and serve.

2 tablespoons ghee or extra-virgin olive oil

4 cloves garlic, minced

1 large onion, chopped

2 medium russet potatoes, peeled and diced (about 3 cups)

3 cups fresh or frozen organic corn kernels

3 cups low-sodium vegetable broth

1½ cups plain unsweetened coconut milk

1 teaspoon minced fresh thyme

1 teaspoon turmeric (optional)

Himalayan or sea salt and freshly ground black pepper

MEAL MATH per serving						
calories	fat	sodium	carbs	fiber	sugar	protein
170	8g	85mg	24g	3g	4g	4g

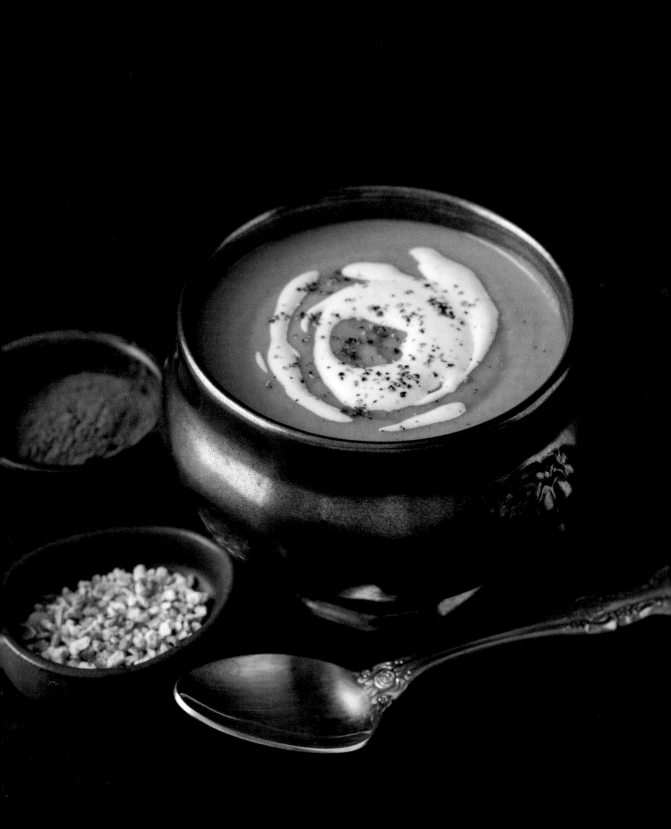

Delight Me:
CURRIED SWEET POTATO

MAKES 8 SERVINGS (SERVING SIZE: 1 CUP)

V Vegan **GF** Gluten-free

My favorite part of Thanksgiving dinner? The sweet potatoes, of course! They're nature's perfect snack food or pre-workout energizer and studies suggest that sweet potatoes may have blood-sugar regulating effects. This is one soup you can be thankful for all year round.

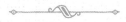

Place the sweet potatoes, broth, coconut milk, apple, nutmeg, ginger, and curry powder into a large pot over medium heat and bring to a boil. Reduce the heat and simmer, uncovered, until apples and sweet potatoes are soft, about 45 minutes. Carefully pour the soup in a high-powered blender and puree until smooth, then return to the pot. Season with salt and pepper to taste and serve.

6 cups sweet potatoes, peeled and chopped (about 5 medium sweet potatoes)

4 cups low-sodium vegetable broth

2 cups plain unsweetened coconut milk

1 large Fuji or Golden apple, peeled, cored, and chopped

1 teaspoon ground nutmeg

1 teaspoon ground ginger

1 tablespoon curry powder

Himalayan or sea salt and freshly ground black pepper

MEAL MATH per serving						
calories	fat	sodium	carbs	fiber	sugar	protein
130	2g	300mg	26g	5g	7g	2g

Recharge Me:
NOT YOUR AVERAGE POTATO SOUP

MAKES 6 SERVINGS (SERVING SIZE: 1 CUP)

V Vegan **GF** Gluten-free

1 tablespoon coconut oil or extra-virgin olive oil

3 cloves garlic, minced

1 small onion, chopped

3 stalks celery, chopped

2 large Yukon Gold potatoes, peeled and diced (about 3 cups)

1 cup dried split green peas, rinsed

6 cups low-sodium vegetable broth

¾ teaspoon smoked paprika, or more to taste

1 teaspoon dried oregano

1 teaspoon dried thyme

⅛ to ¼ teaspoon cayenne pepper

½ teaspoon chili powder

Himalayan or sea salt and freshly ground black pepper

If you believe spuds are duds when it comes to healthful eating, I'm begging you to reconsider this root vegetable. Potatoes contain more potassium than bananas! This hearty, zesty recipe delivers a strong kick and is definitely not your run-of-the-mill potato soup! Give it a shot—just don't blame me when you'll want to make it again (and again and again).

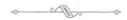

Heat the oil in a large pot over medium heat. Add the garlic and onion and sauté for 3 to 5 minutes, until softened. Stir in the celery, potatoes, split peas, broth, paprika, oregano, thyme, cayenne pepper, and chili powder. Bring the soup to a boil, then reduce the heat and simmer, uncovered, for about 45 minutes to an hour, until the split peas are cooked through and the potatoes are tender. Season with salt and pepper to taste and serve.

MEAL MATH per serving						
calories	fat	sodium	carbs	fiber	sugar	protein
150	2.5g	170mg	28g	5g	4g	5g

Entice Me:
VEGAN TORTILLA SOUP

MAKES 6 SERVINGS (SERVING SIZE: 1 CUP)

V *Vegan* **GF** *Gluten-free*

This soup gives the traditional variation a run for its money. It's the real deal—100-percent all-natural plant-based ingredients that come together for a truly authentic and savory fiesta flavor.

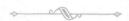

Heat the 1 tablespoon of oil in a large pot over medium heat. Add the onion and garlic and sauté for 3 to 5 minutes, until softened. Stir in the tomato paste and broth. Bring the mixture to a boil, then reduce heat to low and simmer, covered, for about 15 minutes. Stir in the cumin, ¾ teaspoon chili powder, and 2 tablespoons of the cilantro. Add strips from 2 of the tortillas, the tomatoes, beans, zucchini, and jalapeño to the soup. Cover and simmer until the zucchini is tender, 5 to 7 minutes.

While the soup is simmering, preheat the toaster oven to 400°F. Place the remaining tortilla strips on parchment paper, lightly brush them with a touch of olive oil, and sprinkle ¼ teaspoon of chili powder on top. Bake for 10 minutes, or until crispy and lightly golden.

When the soup is done, season with salt and pepper to taste. Garnish the bowls with the remaining 2 tablespoons cilantro and the toasted tortilla strips, and serve.

1 tablespoon extra-virgin olive oil, plus ½ teaspoon more for baking tortilla strips

1 medium onion, chopped

3 cloves garlic, minced

1 tablespoon tomato paste

4 cups low-sodium vegetable broth

¾ teaspoon ground cumin

¾ teaspoon chili powder, plus ¼ teaspoon for baked tortilla strips

4 tablespoons chopped fresh cilantro or chives

4 organic sprouted corn tortillas, sliced into strips

2 Roma tomatoes, chopped

1 cup cooked black beans, no salt added

1 medium zucchini or yellow squash, chopped

1 jalapeño, seeded and minced

Himalayan or sea salt and freshly ground black pepper

MEAL MATH	per serving					
calories	*fat*	*sodium*	*carbs*	*fiber*	*sugar*	*protein*
140	3.5g	120mg	23g	5g	4g	5g

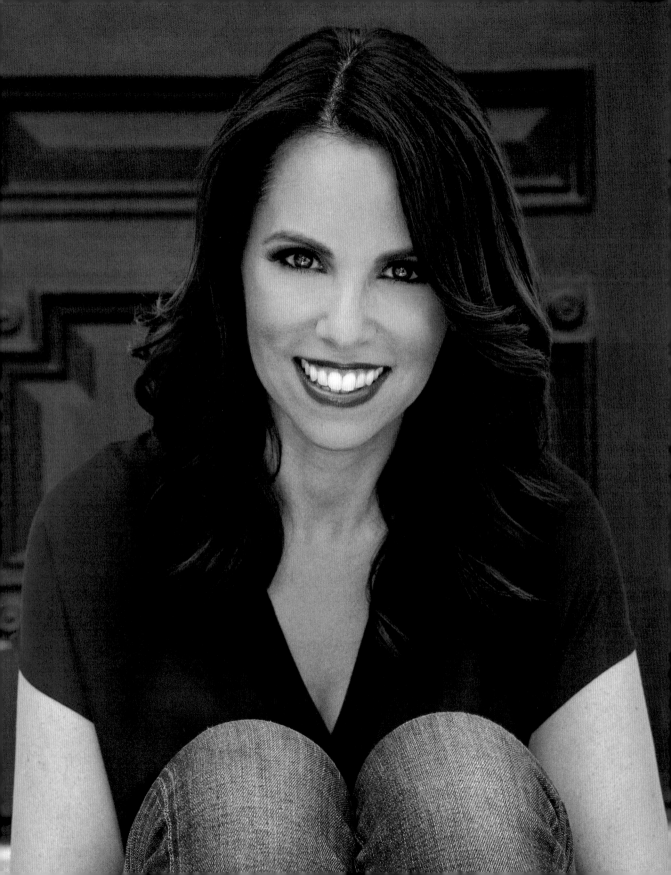

5.

Answer Me

RACHEL ADDRESSES YOUR SOUPING QUESTIONS

No matter how simple and seamless a plan is, having questions is a natural part of the process. Whether you're interested in learning the science behind each spoonful, or need more info on the plan and how to get the most out of it, this Q&A will dish out everything you need to know.

Is there any good research to show that souping helps with weight loss?

Yes, there's tons—that's part of the reason I'm so on board with souping. Here are some studies worth noting:

Research has demonstrated that soup enhances satiety—meaning that it helps fill you up and keeps you feeling satisfied. How? When you incorporate water (or low-cal broth) into a soup, it distributes the nutrients in a way that activates your body's "I'm full" mechanisms. A study in the *Journal of Nutrition* found that blending solids and liquids together suspends tiny bits of nutrients in a manner that stimulates hormones responsible for feelings of satiety, such as cholecystokinin (CCK), glucagon-like peptide-1, and peptide YY. And it does so more efficiently than eating the same foods (and calories) in plated form, even with a glass of water on the side containing an identical amount of liquid.

Research published in the journal *Appetite* found that eating soup not only decreases the number of calories consumed at the next meal by 20 percent, but also that the *type* of soup had no significant effect on calorie intake. In other words, low-cal soups—like the ones in my souping plan—have the same appetite-reducing effects as those that are super high in calories. (I'm looking at you, New England clam chowder.) This has huge implications for weight loss: Souping helps you reduce caloric intake in a way that's genuinely satisfying.

And souping works for the long haul—a study published in *Obesity Research* found that a diet that incorporated two low-cal soups per day over two equal-calorie snacks led to a 50 percent greater weight loss over six months. In this study, the women who included soups in their diet maintained that weight loss over the course of a year. Why? Soups—healthful ones, at least—contain lots of valuable fiber (not a significant source of calories) and water (0 calories!), both of which increase the volume of the meal without causing a big caloric uptick. Soups give you bigger portion sizes, and eating larger amounts of low-calorie foods helps you feel fuller and is key for *sustainable* weight loss. Soup's on—for life!

Is raw produce better than soups—where everything is usually cooked?

Not always. Some vegetables are actually better for you when cooked: Heating them makes certain nutrients more bioavailable. For example, cooking tomatoes breaks down the thick cell walls, improving your body's ability to absorb the potent antioxidant lycopene by up to 35 percent! Carrots, spinach, mushrooms, asparagus, cabbage, and peppers may also have more phytochemicals and antioxidants available for your body to take in when they're cooked compared to when raw. That's why my souping recipes rely heavily on these guys.

Plus, cooking your veg makes it so much easier to get your daily intake of fruit and veg—because many of them shrink down during the process. I mean, who wants to chew 9 cups of raw kale each day? And who can exist on raw produce alone? Salad fatigue is a diet syndrome I see all the time. Souping is a great solution.

One downside of cooking your produce: It may deactivate heat-sensitive vitamin C. But vitamin C is so easy to get in your diet that it's rarely a problem. Plus, I've included plenty of vitamin C–rich fruits and veggies in your *uncooked* breakfast soups and snacks.

If I'm eating "clean," do I even need to think about calories?

Yes—or at least you need to watch your portion sizes (which will do the same thing). I know lots of people claim that you can eat as much as you want and still lose weight—as long as you eat clean. But even clean foods have calories that can affect the size of your waistline.

There's also the belief that diet trends like low carb or gluten-free can help you lose weight without regard to caloric parameters and portion sizes. But once you dig into the details, it's simply not true.

Research shows that when people lose weight on those types of diets, it's not because they cut out one food group or another. It's because restricting the kinds of foods they eat (like not eating carbs or foods that contain gluten) also restricts their overall calorie intake. Calories matter. They just do. Dieters keep looking for a study that will tell them otherwise, but you can't change Science 101.

And that's why I give very specific calorie targets for the clean food snacks in this plan. You need those parameters to succeed. With meals, however, it gets trickier—because there are so many more ingredients and food groups to factor in. I've found that clients have a hard time keeping a mental tally of where they stand calorically while still understanding the necessary components of a whole food weight-loss meal. That's why I developed the Rule of 3. My rules focus on portions and simplicity—which will ensure you get your essential nutrients and keep calories under control without you having to feel like a food accountant. As long as you pay attention to the Rule of 3, you will eat clean and can't go too calorically far afield.

This is *not* to say that "a calorie is a calorie is a calorie." Both the *quality* and *quantity* of what you put into your body matter. Clean calories are better for your health, and I want you to be filling up with calories from real, wholesome foods . . . see the following processed foods question for more.

Why do I need to avoid processed foods?

There are so many reasons to ditch the processed stuff and *get real*.

But first, let's talk about what I mean by *processed*. The term *processed food* technically refers to anything that's been handled by the food industry—which includes things like bagged spinach and precut fruit. Foods that need special handling to make them safe to eat, like pasteurizing milk to remove harmful bacteria, are also considered processed. Even grinding wheat into flour—or nuts to make peanut butter—falls under this broad term.

So if we're going with the technical definition of processed foods, I'm not against all of them. What I *am* against are products with a mile-long list of unpronounceable ingredients added to improve the shelf life, color, or texture. I'm also not a fan of foods that have been unnecessarily or drastically altered from their natural state—like refined grains that have been stripped of their nutrient-rich bran and germ, then bleached, processed, and refortified with manufactured vitamins and minerals. It's *these* things that I refer to as processed foods throughout the book—products that were concocted by some scientist in a lab, not produced by Mother Nature. In general, be on the lookout for familiar ingredients and remember that less is more when it comes to ingredient lists.

Here are some good reasons why you want to avoid these types of processed foods and go for real, whole foods instead:

1. *Processed foods contain additives and chemicals that your body may treat like foreign invaders!* A recent study in the journal *Nature,* for example, found that manufactured ingredients could alter gut bacteria (the all-important microbiome scientists are hot on right now) and cause inflammation that may increase your odds of developing heart disease, diabetes, obesity, and inflammatory bowel disease.

2. *Processed foods are often high in sugar, fat, and sodium.* This trifecta will *not* help with weight loss! Food manufacturers also purposely design these foods to taste irresistible—so you want to eat more, more, more of them.

3. *Processed foods have a lower "thermal effect,"* which means that your body doesn't burn as many calories breaking them down as it does with whole foods, which can also stall weight loss. A 2010 study from Pomona College gave subjects either a "whole" sandwich made with multigrain bread and cheddar cheese or a "pro-

cessed" sandwich made with white bread and a processed cheese product. Both meals contained the same amount of calories, carbohydrates, protein, and fat. Yet the researchers found that the processed meal took *nearly 50 percent* less energy to digest compared to the whole meal, which makes sense because our bodies have to use more energy breaking down complex, fibrous foods compared to their refined equivalents. So, we are burning more calories by choosing real whole foods, which can mean greater success in the weight-loss department.

4. *Not all the calories from whole foods may be absorbed,* which may help slim you down. Research published in the *American Journal of Clinical Nutrition* found that snacking on a small handful of whole almonds may cost you only 129 calories rather than the 170 calories assigned to them. Why? Scientists think the rigid structure in whole almonds may cause some calories to be passed rather than digested. However, this isn't the case with processed forms of nuts—foods such as almond meal and peanut butter will still amount to more calories than their whole-food counterparts. All this to say, research shows that the structure of whole, unprocessed foods may result in lower-than-expected caloric intake! Another reason to get real.

5. *Then there's the fact that whole foods are just more nutritious.* They're packed with fiber, vitamins, minerals, and various phytochemicals that have been shown to protect your cells from damage. While some processed foods add back vitamins and minerals during the manufacturing process, they often don't add *all* of the nutrients—notably, the valuable fiber is often lost. With whole foods, you get the full combination of natural phytochemicals and nutrients in the way nature intended. There's also evidence that some compounds in whole foods interact with one another, providing additional health benefits that a single extracted nutrient may not give you. Plus, research is constantly identifying new phytochemicals and their unique health benefits. We don't yet understand the full spectrum of nutrients that makes a food healthful, but eating real foods is the best way to ensure you are getting the ideal combination. Frankenfoods can't promise that!

Why do I need 30 to 35 grams of fiber a day?

I derived these general targets—30 to 35 grams—after reviewing hundreds of studies on fiber, health, and weight. And there's compelling evidence that fiber works on many fronts to help you drop pounds. For starters, high-fiber foods tend to be low cal yet they bulk up in your system, helping you feel fuller, faster, for fewer calories. (Say that five times fast!) A high-fiber meal also triggers the release of the hormone CCK in your body that *keeps* telling your brain that you're full, so you'll be less likely to get the munchies between meals. And get this: Fiber may actually prevent your body from absorbing some of the calories in the foods you eat.

And let's not forget all the health benefits. There's evidence that high-fiber diets can lower your risk for everything from heart disease and diabetes to breast and colon cancer. Heck, fiber may help you live longer, *period*. The 2012 European Prospective Investigation into Cancer and Nutrition examined the diets of 450,000 men and women and found that those with diets highest in fiber tended to live the longest. In fact, every 10 grams of fiber consumed each day was associated with a 10 percent lower risk of dying from any cause—and it slashed the risk of death from digestive diseases by nearly 40 percent. So get those 30 to 35 grams of *real* fiber daily! Of course, you can go a little over or under— you don't need to obsess over counting grams, but aim for this range.

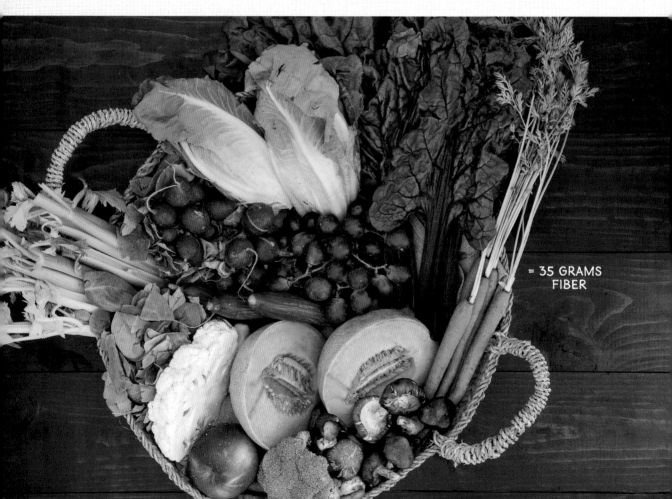

= 35 GRAMS
FIBER

What do you mean by "real fiber?" Is there *un*-real fiber?

Actually, yes. Real fiber, of course, is the kind that occurs naturally in a whole plant or grain. Then there are isolated fibers—like inulin (chicory root), polydextrose, and maltodextrin—that are added to foods by manufacturers. And there may be a difference in terms of how your body treats them. A 2009 study published in the journal *Appetite* compared the satiety of whole apples, applesauce, and apple juice with and without isolated fiber. They found that participants who ate the actual apple before sitting down to lunch wound up eating 15 percent fewer calories than those who ate the fiber-enhanced or processed foods. What this means: Fiber-fortified foods—as well as foods that have undergone processing—may not have the same filling effect that whole, naturally fiber-rich foods do.

Scientists still question whether isolated fibers are as effective at keeping you full, lowering your cholesterol, and managing your blood sugar levels as whole food (non-manufactured) fibers. They don't harm you, but they may not deliver the same benefits. Your best bet is to get the real deal—with real fiber from pure, whole foods.

Why do I need to get at least 10 grams of that fiber at breakfast?

We've all heard that fruits and veggies are rich in fiber, right? And that's true. But you'd actually have to eat a huge basket's worth of produce to get your daily 30 to 35 grams. I've found that the easiest way to meet your fiber goal is to get at least one third of it at breakfast. Then, even if you fall a little short at lunch or dinner, you still won't be wildly under your goal. One of fiber's functions is that it helps you feel full, so a fiberized breakfast is likely to keep you full and minimize cravings throughout the day. The produce at breakfast contributes to your fiber goals and boosts your antioxidant intake—keeping your body running smoothly and minimizing cellular damage.

Why are grains and starches so limited during the 3-Day Restart and 24-Day Transformation—even whole grains?

These parts of the plan are designed to optimize weight loss and teach you a simple strategy to build meals that will deliver maximum weight loss and nutrient content.

Carbs aren't evil—we need them for energy! Technically, carbs include grains, fruits, vegetables, milk, and yogurt. But when we're looking to lose weight and maximize health benefits, we want to choose voluminous and nutrient-rich—yet low-cal—carb options. Fruits and veggies take the spotlight, because not only do they meet these requirements but they're also packed with a variety of phytonutrients.

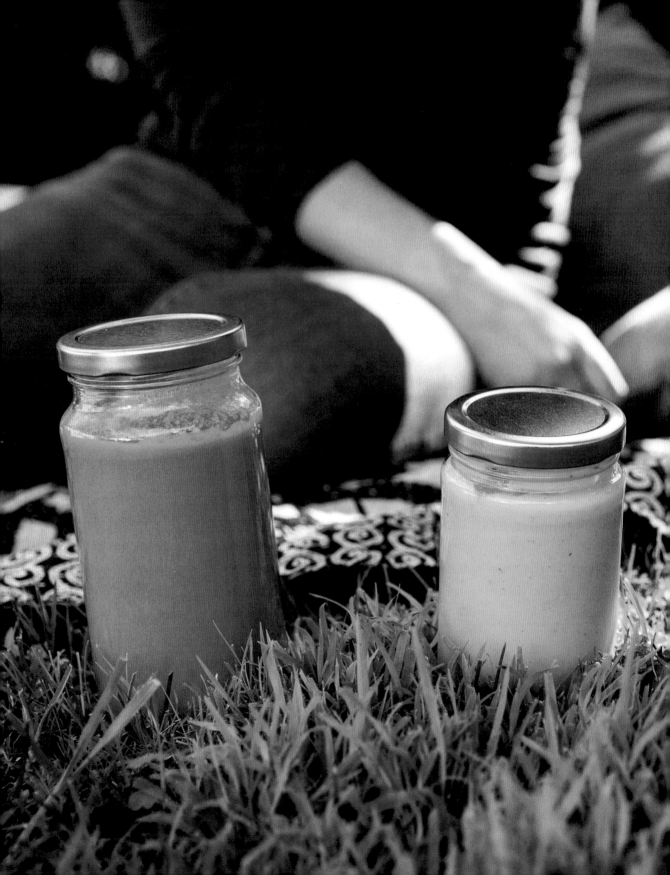

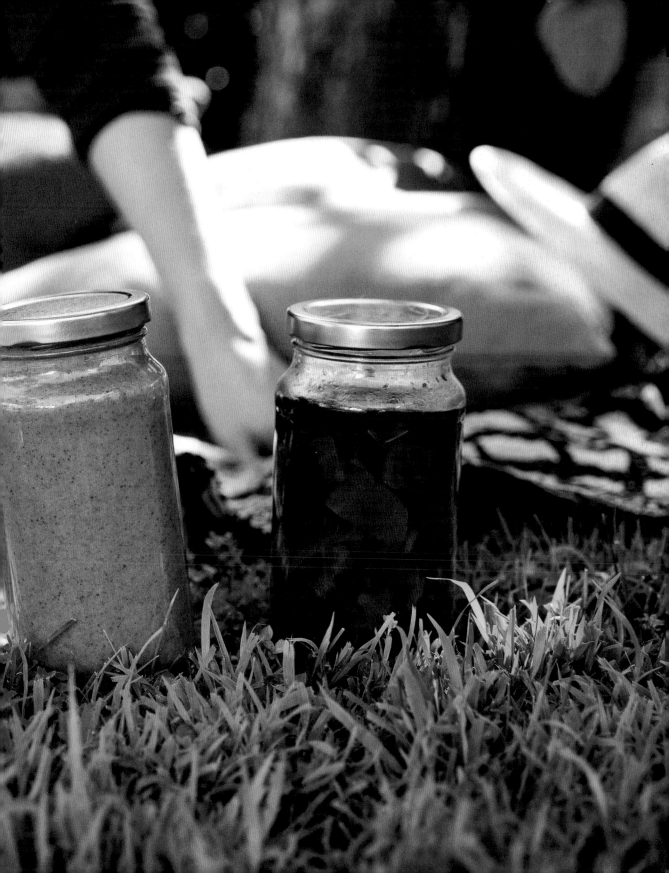

I've learned from years of counseling experience that offering flexibility with grains and starchy vegetables (like potatoes and corn) early on slows down weight loss, not only because these foods have small portions with a high caloric yield but also because they're hard to limit. If the option is there to include them with meals, people often go for it and end up overdoing it.

So while you're on the fast-track weight loss plans, I limit grains and starches to the A.M. This technique is tried, tested, and true—my clients consistently have found it's the easiest, no-brainer way to power up your nutrition and expedite weight loss.

Why are there so many vegan recipes in this book? Do you recommend this type of diet?

Through all my research and practice, I've come to the conclusion that a primarily plant-based diet is the most beneficial for your health. Eating lots of fruits and veg along with plant-based proteins will not only give you the weight loss results you want but will also help you capitalize on the health perks they offer. But I'm not necessarily pushing a full vegan diet—I support but don't entirely follow one. The majority of my diet is vegan, but I choose to eat omega-3-rich, low-mercury fish, occasional organic eggs, and very occasional select organic dairy. This diet is based on my fifteen years of nutrition experience—and it also falls in line with what the American Institute for Cancer Research recommends. I don't completely frown on organic poultry and grass-fed beef and pork—but they just don't have the nutritional advantages of my preferred protein sources.

What's most important for you to grasp regardless of your food philosophy is that anyone who comes through my office doors can improve how they think about what they put in their body, no matter how big or small the modification. Catering to your dietary needs without judgment while keeping the plan realistic and simple is a skill I possess as a nutrition expert and want to carry to you as my readers.

What are the benefits of eating plant-based proteins, like beans and legumes?

I tell my clients to select proteins with benefits to get the most out of their meal. Here's why beans and legumes are some of my top protein picks: They have a super-high fiber content that's great for weight loss, cholesterol levels, cancer prevention, gut health—and, of course, for filling you up. One ¾-cup serving gets you about one-third of the way to your daily fiber goal of 30 to 35 grams. Animal proteins, like chicken and beef, don't have a comparable nutrient profile.

Beans and legumes are also low in fat yet are rich in nutrients including anti-oxidants and essential minerals like copper, folate, iron, magnesium, manganese, phosphorous, potassium, and zinc. And research shows they're also loaded with phy-tochemicals, such as saponins and protease inhibitors—compounds that scientists are investigating for cancer-fighting properties. For example, the famed Nurses' Health Study—which included more than ninety thousand women!—reported a significant association between bean and lentil intake and a reduced risk of breast and colorectal cancer. Animal proteins, on the other hand, don't have phytochemicals with preven-tive health benefits. In fact, they can be pro-inflammatory! They also contribute high levels of saturated fat, which studies have shown elevate the risk and progression of heart disease.

So when you eat plant-based proteins, you're not just getting a hefty dose of fiber and protein—you're getting some mega health perks. Plus, they're much more convenient and wallet-friendly than animal proteins. All solid reasons to jump on the bean wagon!

Soy and tofu pop up in the recipes, but I thought they could increase breast cancer risk. What's the deal?

I get asked about this all the time—people hear that soy increases cancer risk, and often eat more animal-based proteins (such as poultry and meat) instead. But evidence suggests that soy isn't evil. Studies show that eating a moderate amount of soy does *not* increase the risk for breast cancer (or any type of cancer, for that matter)! On the con-trary, research suggests that it may play a *preventive* role in cancer development. Also, eating minimally processed soy like organic tofu and edamame (I'm not talking about soy hot dogs, patties, or protein bars) during childhood and adolescence may provide some protection against breast cancer by encouraging development of healthy breast tissue. Just like any other healthful food, organic soy in moderate amounts (about 5 servings per week) is recommended—and stay close to Mother Nature by avoiding soy-fortified foods.

Soy products are an excellent source of protein, contain beneficial antioxidants, and are a good source of essential minerals—including iron, copper, and potassium. So don't miss out on all these benefits from plant-based protein options like organic edamame, tempeh, and tofu.

My tip: Purchase sprouted, organic tofu—it's not genetically modified, and the pro-cess of sprouting eases digestion and maximizes nutrient absorbtion.

Why do you focus so much on kefir, Greek yogurt, and goat yogurt versus milk? And why organic?

I'm a dairy minimalist. I don't believe you necessarily need to swear off dairy products completely, but because there's so much conflicting information out there, I limit them to the ones that yield the most health benefits: Greek yogurt, goat yogurt, and kefir. These are packed with beneficial probiotics—the "friendly" bacteria that may help optimize digestion and support your immune system. Plus, a 2002 study published in *Cancer Epidemiology, Biomarkers, and Prevention* found that IGF-1—high levels of this hormone have been linked to cancer—may be inactivated when milk is turned into yogurt.

Greek yogurt is super-high in protein that will help keep you satisfied. Goat yogurt is a great alternative if you're allergic to cow's milk—plus, it has more prebiotic oligosacchardies (in amounts similar to human breast milk) that encourage the growth of beneficial gut bacteria. It also may contain more immune-enhancing properties and some people find it easier to digest. My favorite—by far—is kefir. It's smooth, slightly tart, and contains a wider range of digestion-boosting probiotics than yogurt! Studies also suggest that kefir may be the most comfy dairy option for those of you who are lactose intolerant. Of course if you're vegan, there are plant-based alternatives available or you can make your own (see page 139). Regardless, keep dairy to a minimum.

Why do I recommend organic? Because the USDA certifies that the cows aren't given the synthetic hormones rBGH (recombinant bovine growth hormone) or rBST (recombinant bovine somatotropin) to increase milk production. Some research has linked these synthetic hormones with an increased cancer risk. Organic, grass-fed dairy also may be better for you in other ways, too: A study in the *Journal of the Science of Food and Agriculture* found that organic, grass-fed dairy may contain more antioxidants, vitamins, healthful omega-3s, and other beneficial fats than conventional milk, thanks to the cows being grass-fed.

Why 2% Greek yogurt and kefir? Isn't full-fat more in line with "real, unprocessed foods"—albeit more high cal?

There is a trend toward going full-fat with dairy products because they're as close as you can get to unprocessed. Full-fat (a.k.a. "whole") dairy products usually contain 3.5% fat and provide fatty acids like conjugated linoleic acid (CLA), which some studies have linked to lower obesity risk compared to their nonfat counterparts. But the scientific evidence is far from conclusive, so I take a more middle-of-the-road approach. Here's why I recommend 2% dairy (*reduced*-fat), rather than full-fat, low-fat, or nonfat:

1. To lower your hormone exposure. Potentially harmful synthetic growth hormones like rBGH or rBST are stored in milk fat, so when some of that fat is removed, some of those hormones are also taken away. Reduced-fat dairy products may also have lower levels of naturally occurring estrogen and progesterone (which are present even in organic milk), making them a better choice for women at risk for breast cancer, as extra hormones have been shown to increase the odds. The breast cancer specialist in me isn't hopping on the full-fat train because of the potential higher hormone content.

2. To keep calories down. Some studies suggest that full-fat milk is actually associated with reduced body fat compared to low-fat types—in part because the higher fat content may help curb your appetite. Going 2% gives you some of that satiating fat but without the caloric uptick of full-fat dairy. Plus, you can add in other satiating ingredients like avocado, flax, and chia, which boast healthful fat and natural fiber to fill you up without the worry of potentially harmful hormones. I've designed all the recipes in this book to be filling and satisfying on this front: Instead of relying on extra fat to do the job, fiber helps keep you satiated.

3. To still provide you with some of the beneficial CLA, which you wouldn't get in non-fat dairy.

4. To stick with my as-minimally-processed-as-possible mantra. To make nonfat milk, companies mechanically remove the fat, only to add milk solids and vitamins back in through additional processing. 2% milk has *fewer* milk solids added back in than low-fat or nonfat milk, and you're avoiding the excess hormones and calories in full-fat milk—which, by the way, is still processed. 2% is the middle ground.

Do I need to eat fish? Can't I get my omega-3s from plant sources?

I'm sure you've heard about all the health benefits of anti-inflammatory omega-3 fatty acids: A large body of evidence suggests that they can help prevent certain cancers, cardiovascular disease, rheumatoid arthritis, and cognitive disorders. Plus, they may improve skin and hair health and even mood!

But not all omega-3s are the same. The health benefits listed above are mainly linked to docosahexaenoic acid (DHA) and eicosapentaenoic acid (EPA)—fatty acids primarily found in fish and microalgae oil. Plant foods like chia seeds and flaxseeds, on the other hand, have a different form of omega-3s—alpha-linolenic acid (ALA)—that doesn't hold the same potent health benefits as DHA and EPA. Our bodies can convert ALA to DHA and EPA but in *very limited* quantities—I'm talking about between 0.1 to 8 percent for men and 9 to 21 percent for women! That's it.

I'm not saying you should abandon plant-based omega-3s—because the foods that contain them have tons of other benefits. But if you're going for the biggest dose of usable and beneficial omega-3s, choose fish (or microalgae oil, if you're vegan). Aside from helping you lose weight, one of my key dietary goals is to get you to eat health-boosting, anti-inflammatory foods, and DHA and EPA are major players.

Fish oil is readily available in pill form. But here's a quick note about fish oil supplements: The quality and amount of DHA and EPA in fish oil supplements are not regulated and can vary widely. And remember that there are other compounds in fish that are beneficial for your health—like vitamin D, selenium, other good-for-you fatty acids, and protein. While a good fish oil supplement can offer highly concentrated amounts of EPA and DHA, you can get plenty of these by eating three to four servings of low-mercury fish per week. As with everything else, I recommend eating the actual food rather than the pill—and choosing fish in lieu of other animal proteins that are pro-inflammatory and aren't a rich source of omega-3s.

Remind me: What are low-mercury, high-omega-3 sources of fish?

There are lots of options to choose from! Here's a list:

Anchovies	Canned wild albacore tuna (low-mercury brand)	Wild salmon	Shrimp
Atlantic mackerel		Sardines	Trout
Black cod	Canned wild salmon	Scallops	Whitefish

Why are you so in love with matcha? What makes it so great?

When you steep green tea bags, only about 5 to 10 percent of the nutrients end up in the cup (because most of them aren't water soluble). Matcha is distinct from other types of green tea because rather than just steeping the leaves in hot water, the leaves *themselves* are ground into a fine powder. By actually drinking the powdered leaves, you're getting the full power of the polyphenols—compounds with major antioxidant properties and potential weight loss benefits. A study at the University of Colorado found that matcha has up to *137 times greater* concentration of EGCG (a major antioxidant) compared to a normal green tea! I can't think of a better reason to start your morning than with some matcha—think of it as your antioxidant-rich alarm clock.

Additionally, squeezing fresh lemon juice or any type of citrus into your matcha helps maximize your body's absorption of matcha's health-promoting compounds. The key is to buy high-quality 100 percent matcha—it should be a vibrant green color and contain no other ingredients.

I'm having serious sugar/salt cravings! What can I do about it?

I hear this so often as I transition clients to the plan. You may be coming from a place where sweet and salty foods—*intensely* sweet and salty foods—were a staple in your daily life, and your body is just asking for what it's used to. Processed foods in particular are engineered to be high in salt and sugar to keep your taste buds craving more—they're literally created to be addictive. No exaggeration! So when you start cutting back, you can have real withdrawal symptoms. But don't worry. Your palate won't take long to readjust. In my experience, the cravings usually diminish after a couple weeks. Commit to the 3-Day Restart, and as you transition to the 24-Day Transformation, you'll realize that you can use real foods to help satisfy your sweet—or salt—tooth. For example, have one of the dessert soups, or a piece of pure dark chocolate. Or enjoy a date as part of your afternoon snack—it might sound weird, but the natural sweetness will do the trick and satisfy cravings.

As for salt, here's my trick: Add a touch of sea or Himalayan salt to your soups, but do it just at the end of cooking or when you put your plate on the table. If you add salt *during* the cooking process, it binds to the larger protein molecules in your dish, which causes much of the flavor to get lost. Sprinkling it on at the very end, however, gives you a saltier taste while using less salt overall. Win-win.

Can I use sweeteners in these recipes?

Yes, but in moderation—and only natural sweeteners. Think 1 teaspoon raw honey or pure Grade A Dark Color maple syrup. (And no, raw sugar doesn't qualify. It's just sugar with some molasses left in it.) Natural sugar-free replacements, like stevia and monk fruit, are okay, too—but their use should be very limited. As "real" as they may be, a lot of these substitutes are actually sweeter than real sugar, which will only make you crave more intense sweetness in your life. I'm trying to train your taste buds to not desire the extreme sweetness that natural sugar-free replacements offer. We want to scale back on cravings!

Why can't I have alcohol on the 3-Day Restart or 24-Day Transformation?

The Restart and Transformation are meant to give your body a break from having a drink (or 2 or 3) a day. I want to break this cycle, because, first, you're committing to a weight loss regimen—and alcohol has a lot of empty calories. Two glasses of wine, for example, will cost you around 275 calories, and that's if you pour modestly! Second, these plans are all about detox, and alcohol's damage to your liver just doesn't fit the bill. Third, I want you to step back and assess how this habit relates to your personal health history. If there's a strong family history of cancer, you might want to think about scaling back in the long term. I realize that the antioxidants in a glass of red wine can be beneficial for heart disease prevention. If you choose to drink after the 24-Day Transformation, do so in lieu of your evening treat and limit to 1 drink per day for women and 2 drinks per day for men, which is the amount that organizations like the American Cancer Society and the American Institute for Cancer Research allow. However, to really lower your risk for diseases like breast cancer, I recommend limiting yourself to 3 or 4 drinks a week.

I can't buy all organic. What are the benefits of eating organic and what are some of the key foods that are worth getting organic?

When it comes to your health, eating organic is worth investing in. Research suggests that organic fruits and vegetables contain as much as 40 *percent* higher levels of antioxidants and also have greater amounts of beneficial trace minerals. This, coupled with the fact that organic farmers aren't growing crops from genetically modified seeds or using synthetic pesticides and fertilizers, makes me a big fan of choosing organic. Ideally, everyone would buy organic, but that's just not realistic. Because the following fruits and vegetables are prone to having higher levels of pesticide contamination when conventionally grown, I recommend that you opt for their certified organic counterparts:

Apples	Cucumbers	Peaches
Bell peppers	Grapes	Potatoes
Blueberries (domestic)	Hot peppers	Snap peas
Celery	Kale and collard greens	Spinach
Corn	Nectarines	Strawberries
		Tomatoes

On the flip side, here is a list of foods that are the lowest when it comes to pesticide load:

Asparagus	Eggplant	Papayas
Avocados	Grapefruit	Pineapples
Cabbage	Kiwi	Sweet peas (frozen)
Cantaloupe (domestic)	Mangoes	Sweet potatoes
Cauliflower	Onions	

Why do you specify BPA-free containers all the time for items like vegetable broths and canned beans?

BPA, or bisphenol A, is a chemical that's used in the production of "soft" plastics and the linings of some metal products. (If the container has a number 3 or 7 recycle code, it contains BPA.) The chemical can leach from the container into the food inside it—and a growing body of research has linked BPA exposure to detrimental health effects, including impaired brain function, memory and learning, depression, heart disease, type 2 diabetes, breast cancer, and fertility problems. The Food and Drug Administration maintains that very low levels of BPA are safe. But a study by the Centers for Disease Control and Prevention found that nearly every American has BPA in their system—and since we don't know how much it takes to increase your risk for all of these problems, it can't hurt to reduce your exposure. Choosing BPA-free containers is one small way to reduce the risk of a potentially big health concern. To date, I've found that the BPA- and BPS-free (BPS is a chemical that often replaces BPA in packaging) Tetra Paks are a safe container to buy your beans, broth, and plant-based milks in.

How does exercise fit into the plan—and how much exercise should I be getting?

Exercising and maintaining weight loss go hand in hand. In fact, data from the National Weight Control Registry show that out of more than four thousand successful dieters who lost—and kept off—an average of 72 pounds, only 10 percent were able to maintain weight loss without exercise. My take: You've worked so hard, so why gamble to be in that 10 percent?

Plus, exercise has so many added benefits: It revs your metabolism, builds muscle mass (and muscle burns more calories than fat!), relieves stress, and boosts your mood. The recommended amount is at *least* 150 minutes of moderate-intensity exercise (meaning that when exercising you can comfortably talk but not sing) per week—that breaks down to approximately 30 minutes, 5 days per week. But if weight loss is your goal, increasing the amount may lead to quicker results. The key is to find something you love and stick with it!

One word of caution: Just because you're exercising does *not* mean you can eat whatever you like! The point isn't to exercise away high-calorie foods—so don't use food as a reward, as I've seen too many people overeat as a result of this. Unless you're exercising at an intense level for an hour or more for several days a week, you don't need to worry about eating back the calories burned. Otherwise, you don't utilize enough energy during a workout to warrant popping an energy bar or even additional snacks. Just time your meals and snacks around your exercise so you're not running on empty.

I had an off day. What is the best way to get back on track?

Everyone falls off the wagon once in a while. It's important to not beat yourself up—so see each morning as a fresh start. If you're on the 24-Day Transformation, just add an additional day at the end. And keep going—this is a lifestyle! Remember, once you're in the Maintenance phase, it's okay to have those occasional food vacays, just as long as you always come back to my clean-eating basics.

ACKNOWLEDGMENTS

I'm thrilled for the opportunity to thank the special people in my life. I'm truly lucky to be surrounded by so many wonderful and supportive individuals.

A million thank-yous to the following fabulous members of the Beller Nutrition team:

Cassandra Hoo, Cory Ruth, Sam Waranch, and Steph Blank. A very special thanks to Leanna Tu: You're an incredible researcher and in-house editor. You made everything come together and were always ready for a challenge.

To my editor, Deborah Brody, and her assistant, Madeline Jaffe: Thank you for spearheading this project and bringing it to fruition.

To Kris Tobiassen: Thank you for making the interior of this book look amazing.

To the folks at HarperCollins/William Morrow: Thank you for your tremendous support in allowing me to provide an easy and delicious route to those who are looking to forever change the way they think about what they put in their bodies: Liate Stehlik, Lynn Grady, Jennifer Hart, Shelby Meizlik, Anwesha Basu, Molly Waxman, Lucy Albanese, Suet Chong, Rachel Meyers, Anna Brower, and Andrew DiCecco.

This book would not be beautiful without these brilliantly talented and creative individuals:

To Shaun Dreisbash: This book would not have come together without you. Thank you for your organization and writing contributions.

To Freddy J. Nager: Thank you for your creativity, and inspiration as a marketing consultant.

To Teri-Lynn Fisher, who is a food photography genius, and Jenny Park, a food stylist extraordinaire: You both made the food look so good that I could almost eat the pages.

To Nicole Lamotte, for your behind-the-camera talent and ability to capture my family and me in the moment.

To Ariel Fulmer, who is an amazing art director and my go-to for just about anything that needs a stylistic touch: I am amazed by your vision and artistic gifts.

A big thank-you to my agent, Dan Strone, CEO at Trident Media Group. Your enthusiasm, kindness, brains, and hard work made this book a reality. I appreciate your tenacity and support.

To my entertainment attorney, Ken Suddleson. Thank you for always having my back.

I want to give a huge hug and thank-you to my great big family: my mother-in-law, Sheila; my three big brothers; my sisters-in-law, nieces, and nephews. I'm so blessed to have such a loving, supportive, and wonderful family.

To my incredible mother, Shula: Thank you for always believing in me and supporting my dreams. You're my biggest confidant, advice giver, and best girlfriend. To my father, Joe. You have been one of the biggest inspirations for my life's work and mission. I carry you with me always and I miss you so much. You both taught my siblings and me to believe in ourselves and have a work hard, play hard mentality, and you showed us the importance of family and togetherness.

To my beautiful children, Alexia, Jonah, Keira, and Evan: Thank you for your love, humor, honesty, and laughter. Out of all of the hats that I wear, being your mom is the best and most rewarding.

Best for last—my best friend and husband, Mark. I LOVE YOU! You are an amazing daddy to our four kids. You enrich my life and I love always having you by my side. Thank you for supporting and loving me.

UNIVERSAL CONVERSION CHART

OVEN TEMPERATURE EQUIVALENTS	MEASUREMENT EQUIVALENTS *(MEASUREMENTS SHOULD ALWAYS BE LEVEL UNLESS DIRECTED OTHERWISE)*
250°F = 120°C	⅛ teaspoon = 0.5 ml
275°F = 135°C	¼ teaspoon = 1 ml
300°F = 150°C	½ teaspoon = 2 ml
325°F = 160°C	1 teaspoon = 5 ml
350°F = 180°C	1 tablespoon = 3 teaspoons = ½ fluid ounce = 15 ml
375°F = 190°C	2 tablespoons = ⅛ cup = 1 fluid ounce = 30 ml
400°F = 200°C	4 tablespoons = ¼ cup = 2 fluid ounces = 60 ml
425°F = 220°C	5⅓ tablespoons = ⅓ cup = 3 fluid ounces = 80 ml
450°F = 230°C	8 tablespoons = ½ cup = 4 fluid ounces = 120 ml
475°F = 240°C	10⅔ tablespoons = ⅓ cup = 5 fluid ounces = 160 ml
500°F = 260°C	12 tablespoons = ¾ cup = 6 fluid ounces = 180 ml
	16 tablespoons = 1 cup = 8 fluid ounces = 240 ml

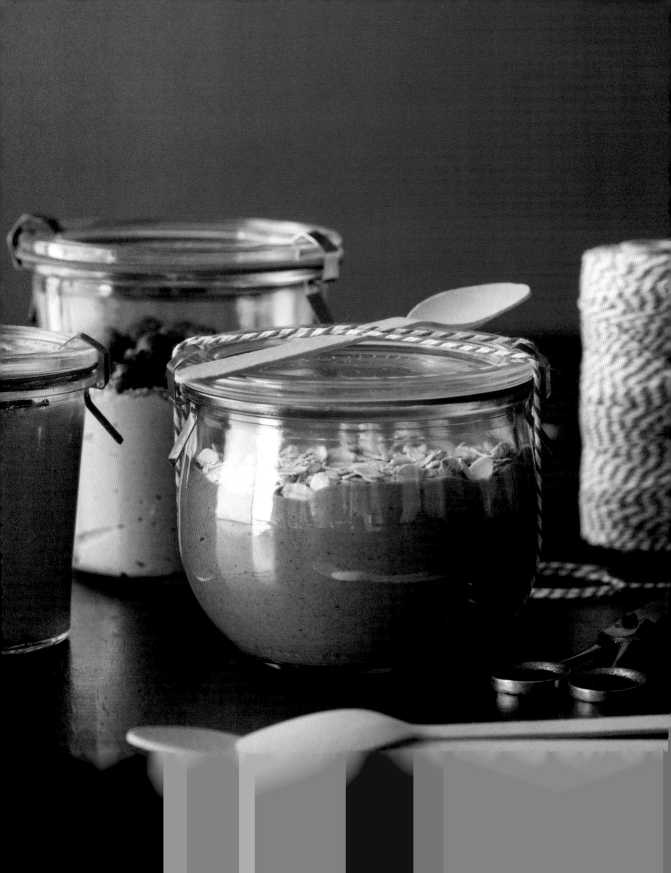

INDEX